SOME LESSER KNOWN HERBAL DRUGS IN AYURVEDA

Indian Medical Science Series No. 53

SOME LESSER KNOWN HERBAL DRUGS IN AYURVEDA

Dr. Gyanendra Pandey

SRI SATGURU PUBLICATIONS
A DIVISION OF
INDIAN BOOKS CENTRE
DELHI-INDIA

Published by:
Sri Satguru Publications
Indological and Oriental Publishers
A Division of
Indian Books Centre
40/5, Shakti Nagar,
Delhi-110007
(INDIA)

First Edition : 1996

ISBN 81-7030-512-8

Published by Sunil Gupta, for Sri Satguru Publications, a division of, Indian Books Centre, 40/5, Shakti Nagar, Delhi-110007, India, and printed at D.K. Fine Art Press, Delhi-110052.

PRINTED IN INDIA

Contents

Acknowledgement : **Dr. V.N. Pandey**, Director, CCRAS, New Delhi

Assistance : **Sumitra Pandey** - Ankur Pandey
478, Aryanagar Colony, Jwalapur-249407
Hardwar, U.P., Phone : (0133) 424270

Dedicated

to

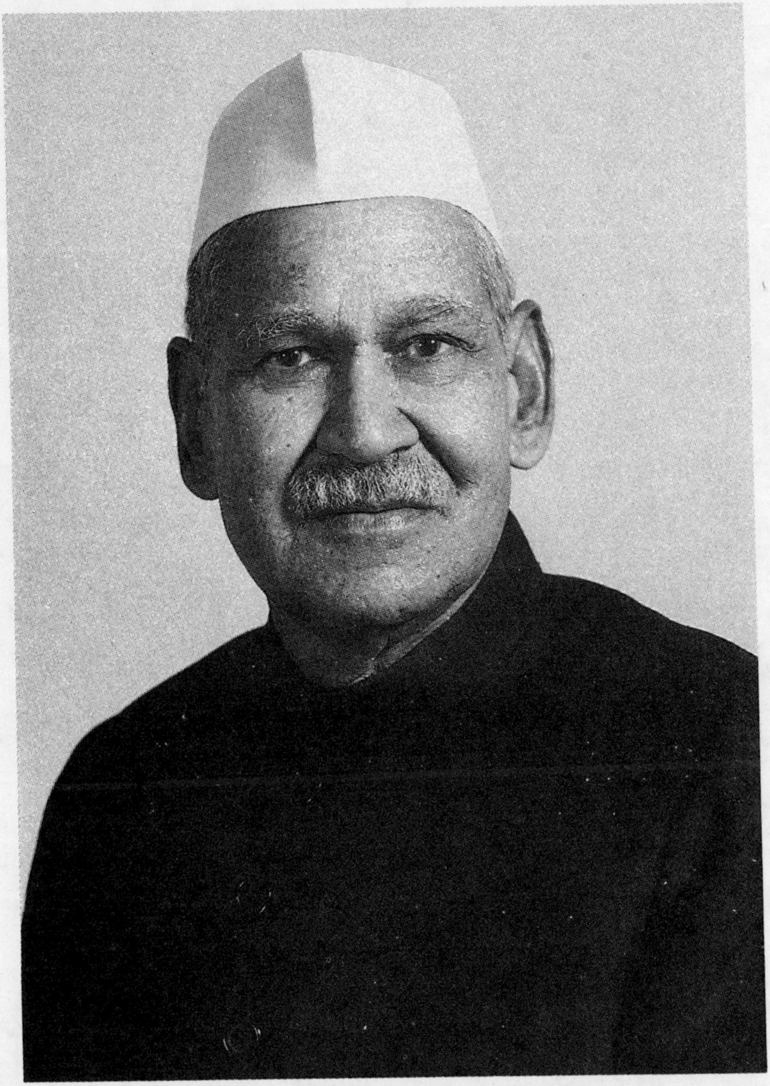

Hon'ble Dr. Shankar Dayal Sharma
His Excellency the President of India

1

Prelude

Project: Multifarious studies on flora of Indian and adjacent regions with special reference to the medicinal potentialities and allied utility, with objectives to provide leads, clues and data supported with ample and multiangled informations on unfamiliar, newer, underexploited and lesser prevalent or acquainted plants, for tapping herbal drug resources, in view to make contribution to the Indian medical science or science of life, the Ayurveda possessing rich treasure of herbal drugs from vegetable sources, for reorientation, revision, supplementation and reviewing of herbal knowledge with scientific approach towards unending search of effective remedies and on-going process of identifying neglected, depleted or extinct drugs through recent advances, current trends and cycles in transformation of herbal knowledge in classical texts, traditions and sciences, in tune with world herbal quest.

Pattern: Material on the plants, mostly wild, in India and adjacent region's, possessing medicinal potentiality with allied utility, by focusing their identification and usefulness as herbal drugs of future paving the avenues for interdisciplinary investigations and detailed studies in medical sciences and therapeusis of Indian medicine in series, by compiling and collating the medicobotanical informations and other various relevant briefs, in a set format mainly comprising botanical names (principal first and synonyms followed), Sanskrit terms; families, regional names, description of taxa, flowering and fruiting season, distribution and occurrence, allied or relevant species, medicinal properties and action, medicinal uses, therapeutic indications, useful parts, other utilities and importance in various purposes, alongwith relevant medicotaxonomical facts on phytodrug sources undertaken in the work, as model in the practicable and integrated manner with co-ordination in botany and medicine, enriching herbal sciences, pioneered by Indian school of learning.

Phytonumarics: The elaboration made on subject dealing with angiospermic flora specifically on plants from natural resources in varied vegetation of country, Indian subcontinent and adjoining countries, possessing significance and relevance to the vistas in focus, presently covers chiefly various medicinally potent and usefully important herbal agents (including vegetable substances), by making reference, incorporation and discussion to different extents and general brevity, which may approximately follow at a glance:

Families	18
Genera	28
Plants Units	28
Species	106
Other species	75
Sanskrit Drug names	140
Regional names	100
Botanical Names	350

Annexures:

Lists and Indices of Families, Genera, Species, Indigenous Drugs, Regional names and Botanical names.

Selected Bibliography

CLASSICAL DICTUM

'अनेनोपदेशेन नानौषधिभूतं जगति किञ्चिद द्रव्यमुपलभ्यते तां तां युक्तिमर्थं च तं तमभिप्रेत्य।'

In the light of this knowledge, there is in the world no substance that may not be used as medicine, in this or that, manner for this or that purpose.

Caraka. Sutra. 26-12

'परीक्ष्यकारिणो हि कुशला भवन्ति।'

Those alone are wise who act after investigation.

Caraka. Sutra. 10-5

'सोयऽमायुर्वेद : शाश्वतो निर्दिश्यते ।'

This science of life- Ayurveds- is declared to be eternal.

Caraka. Sutra. 30-27(I)

'न चैव हयस्ति सुतरमायुर्वेदस्य पारम् ।'

There is no limit at all to the Science of Life.

Caraka. Viman. 8-14

'सोऽनन्तपारं त्रिस्कन्धायुर्वेदम् ।'

The whole science of life, tri-based, extending without end.

Caraka. Viman. Sutra. 1-25

2

Generic Index

Indices with Unit(s) and Component(s) number(s).

Families Index

Species Index

Drugs*

Sūkaparnā	27
Stabamūladalā	27
Sumāḍhipatrā	26
Śākanārī	24
Śalkabahulā	22
Sitāharitapuṣpī	21
Sautracarmā	19
Ṛjukaṇṭā	21
Saumanasyā	17
Sujātā	16
Sitapuṣpā	15
Sautrikā	11
Sunetrā	8
Supuṣpā	5
Sandhānikā	4
Trikaṇṭakā	23
Tiktaviṭapa	15
Tūladharā	6
Tiktaparnī	5
Trikoṇabīja	4
Tamapriyā	1
Tvacyā	20
Vṛntapatrā	22
Vikṣatā	16
Viṣamapaksikā	10
Vṛntikā	8
Vāmikā	6

---

*Model Sanskrit names with pentaterms integrating single drug mostly relevant to principal source plant indicated with number in order.

3

Plants Units

1. Ropaṇapatrikā-Adhāramulā-Maśakagranthiphalā-Tamapriyā

A1.Adenostemma lavenia (Linn.) O.Kuntze.

Adenostemma viscosum J.R. & G.Forst.

Verbesina lavenis Linn.

Adenostemma lavenia (L.) O.Kurtze. var, **elata** Kitamura.

A. latifolium D. Den.

Asteraceae

Seh-bythrit

Annuals. Stems decumbent and rooting at base, ascending upwards, glabrous or glabrescent downward, glandular-hairy upward. Leaves ovate-lanceolate or oblong, obtuse, acuminate or acute, attenuate or narrowed to the base into a subulate petiele, subglabrous, 2-7 (-10) × 1.5-5 cm. Heads 0.6 × 0.4-0.5 cm., in lax cerymbs. Cerella 0.1-0.15 cm. long. Style-arms 0.25 cm. long.

July or August to November; October to January.

Throughout India ascending the Himalayas and other ranges.

1.1*Adenostemma lavenia* (L.) O.Kurtze Erect rarely decumbent annual glabrous, pubescent or viscidly pubescent. Leaves sessile or petioled, opposite or the upper alternate, broadly ovate or cerdate, nearly glabrous, serrate. Heads few or many, on lax or dense panicles or corymbs, homogamous receptacle flat, marked; corolla all equal, tubular, regular, tube short, limb campanulate, 5-teethed; bracts obtuse, 5-ribbed, sparingly warted, pappus hairs 3-5, short, rigid, often clavate inserted in a short ring.

Common in damp, shady localities, sal forest and forest clearings in Siwalik region (Dehradun, Uttar Pradesh).

1.2 *Adenostemma lavenia* (L.) Kuntze. Glabus or hairy annual herb. Leaves 6-22 X 4-14 cm., broadly ovate, acute, cuneate below, glabrescent. Involucral bracts glandular-hairy. Corolla and style arms white. Achenes tuberculate; pappus knobs 3-4.

Asiatic now Pantropical. Common in Ghats ans western plains, usually in shaded moist places, Karnataka state in Southern India.

1.3 *Adenostemma macrophyllum* (Bl.) DC. *Adenostemma macrophyllum* Bl. (*pro. syn.*)

Asteraceae

Annual-perennial, decumbent-ascending, herbs. Stems often rooting below, glandular-hairy at the top, lower down glabrous. Leaves ovate-lanceolate to oblong, obtuse or acute, with a narrowed base, serrate in the upper part, slightly rugose, glabrous, 5-15(-20) X 2-10 cm. Heads 0.8-1 cm. across, in many-headed corymbs. Peduncle 0.5-1.5 cm. long. Involucre 0.5-1 cm. long, with oblong subspatulate, ciliate bracts, Corolla 0.25-0.3 cm. long, with a campanulate, fomentose limb. Style-arms 0.35 cm. long. Achenes oblong, slightly curved, glandular-hairy at first, smooth, 0.3 cm long. Pappus of 2-4-0. cm. long setae.

July to November.

Common in marshy localities, cascades and watercourses in Siwalik region (Dehradun, Uttar Pradesh).

1.4 These two species are quite distinguishable. For the instance, the smooth achenes, larger involucres, bigger heads, and longer corollas separate *Adeneostemma macrophyllum* (Bl.) DC from *A. lavenia* (Linn.) O.Kuntze. characterized by the tubercluate achenes, shorter involucres, smaller heads and shorter corollas alongwith other features.

Comparatively the achenes smooth, involucres 0.5-0.6 cm. long, heads 0;.8-1 cm. long, corolla 0.25-0.3 cm. long, tomentese in the upper part are in *Adeneostemma camrophyllum* (Bl.) DC; whereas *A. lavenia* (Linn.) O.Kuntze is with achenes tuherculate, involucres 0.3-0.4 cm. long, heads 0.6 cm. long, corolla 0.1-0.15 cm long and lanate in the upper part.

1.5 Various species alongwith their varieties of Adenostemma Forst. follow, for the instance:-

Adenostemma lavenia var.. *angustifolium* (Cl.) Kester.

A. lavenia var.. *elatum* (D. Don.) Hochr.

A. lavenia var. latifolium (D. Don.) Panigrahi

A. lavenia (Linn.) Kuntze. var. *lavenia*

A. lavenia var. *madurehse* (DC) Panigrahi

A. lavenia var. microcephyllum (DC) Kester.

A. lavenia var. reticulatum (DC) Panigrahi

A. lavenia var. rugosum (DC) Rl.

1.6 *Adenostemma microphyllum* (Bl.) DC is sometimes treated earlier as synonymous to *A. viscosum* var. *parviflorum* (Bl.) Hook.f.; and later recognised as distinct species. Remarkable differences constantly maintain it a distinct species, and hence two species are referred of Adenestemma J.R. & G. Forst.

1.7 Various parts and whole plants of Adenostemma J.R. & G. Forst. are medicinally useful.

Leaves of *Adenostemma lavenia* (L.) Kuntze. are considered useful as antiseptic. Juice is considered as a stimulant and aternutatory. Leaves are applied after grinding and making a paste over wounds, cuts and injuries, insects bites and also bruises. Fresh juice is also externally applied over cuts and similar conditions. Leaves paste or juice is considered useful against poisonous insects bites or stings as well as in injuries and wounds

2. Himāmlikā - Raktaphalā - Anupaspā - Udarahitā

A2.*Antidesma acidum* Retz.

Antidesma diandum Retz.

A. diandrum (Rexb.) Roth.

A. ghaesembilla sensu Hook.f.

A. acidum Retz. non Gaertn

Stilago diandra Rexb.

A. lanceolaria Rexb.

Euphorbiaceae

Kali-khatai (U.P.; Siwalik), Dhokki (Oudh), Amli (Hindi), Amli. Imli, Amari (Hindi), Malta (Bengal), Sana Kulipa (Kannada),

Manchi palleri (Telugu), Kinbalia (Burmese), Laphasakho (Mech.), Aburak (Garo), Geri-ambal (Jharua), Chhothahelach (abuteggo), Nekhon-tenga (Jharma) (Assam), Dieng-japeu, Chouding (Khasi), Son-karancha (Sylhet), Ing-sum-aring (Mik.)

Deciduous shrub or small tree; branches spreading; young parts rusty-pubescent. Bark greyish brown, thin rough; blaze light red. Leaves turning deep red before falling, 1.5 by 0.5-1.5 in., variable, oblong to lanceolate, ovate inobovate, acute or acuminate, entire, sub-coriaceous, glabrous and shining above, rusty pubescent along the nerves beneath; lateral nerves 3-8 on either half; base cuneate or acute; petiole 0.5-1.5 in. long, pubescent, stipules lanceolate, deciduous. Flowers minute, dioecious; all flowers pedicelled. Male flowers calyx obtuse, 4- lobed or obscurely 4- toothed, stamens 2 (rarely-3) at the base of the glabrous disc, pistillode O. Female flowers calyx more deeply lobed than the males; disc anular. Ovary glabrous, style terminal. Fruit about .16-.2 in. across, smooth, purplish, red when ripe, ovoid, acute.

Summers to cold seasons; May-June to December-January

Outer ranges of Himalaya from Garhwal and Kumaon eastwards; also in Bengal and in Central, Western and Southern India, extending to Ceylon and Burma. Common throughout the Assam province.

2.1 *Antidesma diandrum* Reth. Small deciduous or shrub-bush, the young parts usually glabrous outer bark smooth, grey. leaves bright green, turning red before falling, thin shortly petioled, varying in size from 1 to 6 in. in length, lanceolate or ovate-lanceolate, acute or acuminate, glabrous above, rarely pubescent beneath; stipules linear, acute, about twice as long as the petieles. Flowers minute, all pedicelled, in long slender glabrous, or pubescent racemes; bracts ovate, shorter than the pedicels. Male and female flowers. Drupes 1/6 in. diam., purplish-red when ripe.

Common in the forests of Siwalik range (Dehradun and Saharanpur districts), and eastward along the Sub-Himalayan tracts of Rohilkhand, South Oudh and eastern U.P. area bordering Nepal. (Gorakhpur district).

2.2 *Antidesma diandrum* Roth. A large shrub of small tree, deciduous, glabrous or branchlets rusty-pubescent. Leaves thin, lanceolate or elliptic-lanceolate, base acute, blade up to 5, pétiole

1/5 in., stipules deciduous. Racemes lax, slender, often simple, quite glabrous; fls. all pedicelled; calyx 4 - lobed. Stamens 2, rarely 3, at the base of the small glabrous disk. Fruit 1/6 in. diam., purplish red, edible. Leaves turning brick-red before falling.

Sub-Himalayan tract from Jumna eastwards; common in sal forests, Bihar, Chhota Nagpur, Central Provinces, Western Pininsula, Assam ascending up to 45,00 ft. Manipur, Bengal, Burma, lower and upper-Ceylon.

2.3 *Antidesma ghasaembilla* Gaertn.

Antidesma pubescens Roxb.

A. paniculatum Roxb.

Euphorbiaceae

Aburak, Amrul, Acchal, Chamtu, Khatua, Mathasur, Nunnuniya; Umtae (Hindi and Punjabi), Khudijamb (Bengla), Jhondri (Madhya Pradesh), Lona (Telugu), Janupulisaru (South.)

Small deciduous tree, with greyish bark; branchlets pubescent or fulvous-tomentose. Leaves 2-4 in, long, oval obovate or orbicular -oblong, rounded or emarginate at the apex, glabrous or nearly so on the upper surface, pubescent or tomentose beneath; base rounded or subcordate; main laeral nerves 5-6 pairs; petieles 1/4-1/2 in., long; stipules about as long as the pedicels, lanceolate, acute, downy. Flowers greenish-yellow, sessile, arranged in slender panicled spikes. Male flowers calyx 5-7 partite, densely fulvous-hairy; stamens 4-7, anthers crescent-shaped; disk 5-part., pubescent. Female flowers calyx as in the male fl.; disk annulate; ovary hairy; stigmas minute, recurved. Drupe subglobose when fresh, about 1/3 in. in diam., reddish or black when ripe.

May to June; March-may to colder months.

Outer Himalayan ranges at low elevations, from the Sutlej to Bhutan; also in Assam, Bengal and from Central, western and Southern India to Ceylon; extending to Burma, the Andamans, the Malay Paninsula and Islands. China and Australia.

2.4*Antidesma ghaesembilla* Gaertn. Small deciduous tree or shrub; young shoots rusty or brown tomentose; branchlets lenticellate. Bark light brown furrowed, somewhat corky. Leaves 1.5-3 by 1.2 in., ovate, oblong, broadly elliptic or subrobicular, rounded or obtuse, bluntly or shortly acuminate, entire, coriaceous, glabrescent or pubescent along the nerves above, pubescent or tomentose beneath; lateral nerves 5-7 on either half arching, sub-parallel, base rounded, truncate or sub-cordate; petiole .1-.5 in. long; stipules caducous, linear-lanceolate, tomentose. Flowers minute, in densely, pubescent terminal and axillary much branched spikes. Male flowers sessile, yellowish green; segments ovate, 5-7 partite, densely woolly tomentose; stamens 4-7; disc 5-partite, pubescent minute. Female flowers sub-sessile, disc annular, pilose, ovary densely pubescent; stigmas recurves. Drupe sub-globose, about .2 in. long, red ultimately purplish, black when ripe.

Assam province; Goalpara, Kamrup, Newgong, Sibsagar, Sylhet, Cachar, Khasi and Jaintia Hills, up to 2,800 ft. elevation areas in state and adjoining areas.

2.5 *Antidesma ghaesembilla* Gaertn. A small deciduous tree; branchlets, petioles, young leaves and inflorescence usually soft-tomentose, rarely glabrous. Leaves broad-elliptic, sometimes obovate, mostly obtuse, blade 2-4 pet. about 3/4 in., stipules horse, stipules early deciduous. Flowers in sessile in slender panicled spikes, stamens 4-7, anthers horse-shoe shaped, disk 5-lobed, pubescent. Ovary pubescent; fruits red to black, small.

Tropical Himalayas from Simla to Bhutan, in Konkan and North Kanara. Common in the Sub-himalayan tract forests of Rohilkhand, North Oudh and eastern U.P. area adjacent to Nepal; Sarda eastwards.

2.6 *Antidesma bunius* Spreng.

Eupherbiaceae

Malung-renu (Tipp.), Karanda (Sylhet), Bol-aborak (Gare), Dieng-sah-silli (Khasi), Son-kong-asing (North-east Frontier Tract), Amati (Marathi), Nolalati (Tamil), Anepu (Telugu), Nulitali (Marathi), Himalchari (Nepal).

Small evergreen tree; shoots tomentose. Leaves variable, elliptic-oblong, lanceolate, obovate or oblanceolate, acuminate or acute, 7.5-1.5 cm., nerves 6-12 pairs, arched; petiole short; stipules ovate-cordate, deciduous. Spikes simple or panicled, stout, pubescent, villous or tomentose often 10-13 cm. long. Flowers about 0.2 mm. across (rather large for the genus); male flowers in pdeuncled lax spikes; female flowers in recemes, both up to 13 cm. long; disk of male flowers lobed, of female cupular, Drupe about

6 mm. long, ellipseid, compressed, red, ultimately black, when ripe.

April-May to August.

Throughout the hotter parts of India from Nepal and Sikkim Terai and Assam southwards to Singapore and from Parasnath (Bihar) to Ceylon and Malaya Islands.

2.7 *Antidesma bunius* Spreng.

Small evergreen tree of 30 to 36 ft. height; young parts hairy. Bark dark-brown, .16 in. thick; fibrous and pinkish-brown inside. Leaves 2-7 by 1.5-5 in., oblong-lanceolate, lanceolate, oblanceolate or oblong-elliptic, shortly acuminate obtuse, often mucronate, entire, coriaceous, glossy green, glabrescent; lateral nerves 5-10 on either half, arcuate; petiole .1-.4 in. long, pubescent; stipules caducous, reddish.

Flowers about .1 in., across, in simple, or racemose pubescent spikes; bracts minute. Male flowers calyx cupular, shortly teethed, sparsely pubescent; disc glabrous, lobed, fleshy; stamens 3; pistillode dilated at the top. Female flowers calyx truncate or sub-entire, persistent in fruit; disc cupular, glabrous; overy glabrous; stigmas 3-4, small.

Fruit .25 in. long, ellipsoid, compressed, red, ultimately blackish (pedicelled up to .2 in. long).

Subhimalayan tract from Nepal eastwards, ascending to 3,000 ft., Assam, Khasi hills, Manipur, Chhota Nagpur, Western Ghats, Upper Burma, Arakan Yoma 3-4,000 ft., Ceylon, China, Malaya Archipelago.

2.8*Antidesma bunius* Spreng. A small evergreen tree, youngest shoots hairy; leaves glabrous, elongate-elliptic or elliptic-lanceolate, acuminate; flowers spikes pubescent, male simple, female often compound, calyx of female usually hairy, sometimes glabrous, ciliate on margin; anthers 3, male fls. shortly pedicelled; fruits 1/3 in. diam., very juicy, red, turning black when ripe.

Assam province; Sylhet, Garo hills, Sibsagar, North-east Frontier Tract, Lakhimpur, North Cachar hills, Lushai Hills, Manipur, Khasi and Jaintia Hills.

2. 9*Antidesma acuminatum* Wall.

Euphorbiaceae

Dieng-seh-lang-ngiu (Khasi), Pani-helech (Assam), Dieng-pothar (Khasi hills).

Shrub or small trèe; branchlets tomentose. Leaves bifarious, 2,5-9 by 1.3 in., elliptic-lanceolate or oblong, lanceolate, caudate-acuminate, entire, thinly coriaceous, almost glabrous, except the midrib and nerves beneath; lateral nerves 6-11 on either half, slender, arching; base rounded or obtuse, sometimes unequal-sided; petiole .1-.3 in. long. Male flowers in panicled hairy racemes; sepals 3-4; disc fleshy, glabrous; stamens 3-4; pistillode conspicuous. Female flowers in much larger panicled racemes; ovary glabrous. Fruits .16 in. long, red when ripe, ultimately blackish, ellipsoid, acuminate, crowned by the style.

June-July to November-January; Summers to Winters

Eastern Himalayan region, Sikkim foot hills, ascending to 3,000 ft., Assam, Khasi hills, Chhota Nagpur.

2.10*Antidesma acuminatum* Wall. A large shrub, branchlets, petioles, stipules and midrib of leaves tomentose; leaves shining above, elliptic-lanceolate, blade 4-12, petioles up to 1/5 in. long; male flower racemes 2-6 in. long, mostly panicled, rachis and bracts densely hairy, pedicels, longer than bracts, calyx of 4 broadly ovate sepals, glabrous or hairy stamens 3-4; female flowers sometimes with short stamens; fruits 1.6 in. long, acuminate.

Assam province; Lakhimpur, Newgong, Sylhet, Sibsagar, Khasi and Jaintia hills up to 4,000 ft.

2.11 *Antidesma khasianum* Hook.f.

Euphorbiaceae

Dieng-seh-syilih (Khasi)

Shrub or small tree; young shoots sparsely pubescent, branching-branchlets greyish-white. Leaves bifarious, 2-6 by 1.2-5 in., oblong-elliptic, elliptic-lanceolate or narrow-lanceolate, acuminate, entire, sub-ceriaceous, darka green above, midrib and nerves sparingly pubescent when young, otherwise glabrous. Lateral nerves 6-10 cm. on either half; slender, arched; base cuneate or acute; simple linear-lanceolate;petole 1-3 in. long. Male flowers skender, pubescent, up to 2 in. long, flowers pedicelled; calyx cupular, shortly 3-4 lobed; stamens 2-4, inserted in the disc. Female flowers racemes much storter. Fruits subglobose or ellipsoid, .23-3 by .12-16 in., red, ultimately blackish, crowned with remains of the style; stone strongly reticulated.

July to November

South Deccan, Peninsula, Ceylon, Eastern Himalayan region.

2.12 *Antidesma khasianum* Hook.f. A large shrub. Young shoots and inflorescence hairy, otherwise glabrous. Leaves shape from elliptic-lanceolate to linear-lanceolate, blade 2-7, petioled; male racemes hairy, lax about 1 in. or more long; calyx glabrous, cupular, shortly 3-4-lobed, stamens 2-4; fruits about 1/2 in. long, tipped by the 2-3 rigid bases of stigmas.

Assam province, Cachar and Khasi hills, Lakhimpur, Sylhet and Jaintia hills, up to 47,00 ft. elevation.

2.13 *Antidesma manasu* Miq.

Euphorbiaceae

Trees up to 10 meters; shoots pubescent. Stipules large, ovate-lanceolate, subpersistent; leaf blade 12-20 by 3-7 cm. oblong-lanceolate, acute to acuminate, rounded below, glabrous Flowers. Flowers pedicelled. Calyx lobes 4, hairy. Stamens 5, inserted on hollows of disc. Drupe somewhat oblique oblong tipped by stigmas, 1-seeded, turning red with age.

December to August.

Western Peninsular India. Common in Ghats along margins of wet deciduous and semi-evergreen forests, Karnataka.

2.14 *Antidesma roxburghii* Wall.

Stilago tomentoso Rexb.

Eupherbiaceae

Shrub; young branches densely rusty-villous. Leaves 4-9 by 2-3 in., obovate or oblong, elliptic-acuminate, entire, sub-coriaceous, puberulous above, villous tomentose beneath; lateral nerves 8-10 on either half; base rounded, often unequal; petiele .05-.15 in.; stipules persistent. Flowers sessile in stout spikes, 4-6 in. long. Calyx 3-4 partite, villous, segments rounded. Stamens 3-4; disc glabrous; pistillode sub-globose. Female flowers disc hairy; ovary tomentose. Fruit about .25 in. long, ovoid or ellpsoid.

Summers to cold seasons.

Assam province, Sibsagar, Sylhet.

2.15 *Antidesma nigricans* Tulasne

Eüphorbiaceae

Shrub with tomentose branches. Bark brown. Leaves 3.5-7 by 1-2.5 in., elliptic-lanceolate or oblong-lanceolate, acuminate, entirem sub-coriaceous, glabrous, the midrib above and beneath pubescent; lateral nerves 6-12 on either half arcuate, joined by intramarginal nerve; base obtuse, sometimes unequal; petiole .05-.02 in. long, tomentose. Male flowers sessile. Calyx 4-partite. Disc glabrous, hemispheric. Stamens 4, inserted on the disc. Ovary glabrous; disc glabrous; stigmas terminal. Fruit ovoid, .16 in. across.

October to November and other months.

Assam province, Sibsagar, Sylhet.

2.16 Some other species of genus *Antidesma* Linn. may also be referred in this context:-

Antidesma wattii Hook.f.

A. volutinosum Blume.

A. volutinum Tulasne.

A. martabanicum Presl.

A. cuspidatum Muell.-Arg.

A. fruticulosum Kurz.

A. mortizil Muell.-Arg.

A. coriaceum Tul.

Embellia non lucida Wall ex DC.

A. lucidum Merr.

A. fallax Muell.-Arg.

2.17 Various species of *Antidesma* Linn. may be distinguishable by different features. For the instance, the leaves very obtuse, flowers sessile, stamens 4-7 and ovary hairy in *Antidesma ghaesembilla* Gaertn.; whereas *Antidesma diandrum* Reth. with leaves acute or acuminate, flowers pedicelled, stamens usually two and ovary glabrous.

Broadly the species of *Antidesma* L. are grouped for characteristic distinction. Ovary tomentose in *Antidesma ghaesembilla* Gaertn., *A. roxburghii* Wall, *A. volutinosum* Blume. and *A. halferi*

Hook.f.; and the ovary glabrous in rest of relevant species, which are distinguished by specific floral characters. Male flowers sessil and calyx not deeply lobed in *Antidesma bunius* Spreng.; male flowers sessile but calyx deeply 4-lobed in *Antidesma velutinum* Tulasne., *A. cuspidatum* Muell. -Arg., *A.nigricans* Tulasne.; and male flowers pedicelled in other species viz. *Antidesma diandra* Roth.; *A. khasianum* Hook.f., *A. morttzil* Muell.-Arg., *A. acuminatum* Wall., *A. menasu* Miquel. and *A. maratabanicum* Presl.

The species having male flowers pedicelled, calyx obtuse, 4-lobed, female calyx deeply 4-lobed are separated by particular characters in calyx, stamens and leaves mainly. Leaves 1-5 in. long and stamens 2 (very rarely 3) in *Andidesma diadrum* Roth.; calyx segments broadly ovate, four and leaves 3-10 in., stamens 3-4 in *A. acuminatum* Wall.; calyx cupular, shortly 3-4 lobed, leaves 2-7 in. and stamens 2-4 in., *A. khasianum* Hk.f.; calyx 3-4-partite, leaves 3-5-8 in. and stamens 3-4 in *A. menasu* Miq.; and calyx cupular, unequally 4-lobed, leaves 1.5-4 in and stamens 3-4 in *A. wattii* Hook.f. Similarly the species having male flowers sessile may be distinct. Calyx cupular, very shortly 4-lobed, leaves 2-6 in. long, glabrous and stamens 3 in *Antidesma bunius* Spreng; and calyx 4-partite, leaves 3-5-7 in. and stamens in *A. nigricans* Tulasne.

Antidesma Linn. in Euphorbiaceae is sometimes included under Stilaginaceae or Antidesamceae. *Antidesma acidum* Retz. keeps *Antidesma diandrum* Roth. and also *A. ghaesembilla* Gaertn. as synonyms. Likewise *Antidesma bunius* Spreng. stands with *A. thwaitesianum* Muell.-Arg.

2.18 *Antidesma diandrum* Roth. A deciduous shrub, 5-15 ft. high with stems up to 6 in. diam. Bark brown, fairly smooth, thinly mealy-corky, blaze .2-.3 in., cheasy, not fibrous, pink, with or without whitish bands and tinged with chlorophyll outside. Leaves 2-6 by 1-2 inches, variable, the larger, the larger usually oblong-lanceolate, the smaller obovate or elliptic, usually acuminate, base acute, glabrous above, glabrous or slightly pubescent beneath, rather thick, nerves faint. Petiole .1-.2 in. long. Flowers beneath, greenish, subsessile, in slendererminal recemes 1-2.5 in. long; racemes simple or with a few branches. Stamens usually 2. Drupes ovoid, .2-.25 in. long, succulent, turning first red and finally black.

Plant occurring throughout the area up to 5,000 ft.; and fairly common in sal and miscellaneous forests of the sub-Himalayan tract and outer hill region, Kumaon ranges, Uttar Pradesh hills. The leaves which are acidic, turn pink or dull red sometimes before falling, and brightly coloured leaves seen from December to March; flowers during May to June and fruits in colder months or December to January.

2.19 *Antidesma ghaesembilla* Gaertn. A deciduous shrub or small tree. Bark pale, smooth or slightly cracked. Blaze pink. Leaves 2-4.5 in. long, oval obovate or orbicular, oblong, rounded or emarginate at the apex, sometimes also with a short blunt acumen, glabrous or nearly so above, pubescent or tomentose beneath; base rounded or subcordate; main lateral nerves 3-6 pairs. Petiele 2-5 in. long. Flowers greenish-yellow, small, subsessile, in densely tomentose panicled racemes 1-2 in. long. Stamens 4-7. Dupe subglobose, .2 in. diam., reddish or black when ripe.

Plant occurring occasional or scattered in Kumaon region at lower elevation, Terai or Bhawar region; mostly indry localities up to 2,000 ft. in Uttar Pradesh hills. It flowers during May to June or summers.

2.20 Both species of *Antidesma* Linn. in Uttar Pradesh hills and foothills e.g., Kumaon region, may be distinguishable. Leaves acute or acuminate and flowers in glabrous usually simple racemes in *Antidesma diandrum* Roth.; whereas *A. ghaesembilla* Gaertn. is with leaves rounded at the tip and flowers in sometimes panicled racemes.

2.21 Various species of *Antidesma* Linn. are medicinally useful and utilised in allied purposes.

The fruits of *Antidesma ghaesembilla* Gaertn. are edible. Fruits of *A. diandrum* Roth. are edible, and the leaves are acid and made into preserve. Fruits of *A. bunius* Spreng. are edible. The acid leaves of *A. diandrum* Rexb. are eaten, and the fruit of this species are also acid and eaten. Like wise the fruits of *Antidesma khasianum* Hk.f. are edible. The acid fruits as well as the leaves are eaten under the uses of *A. ghaesembilla*. Similarly the acid fruits, leaves and small reddish fruits have a pleasantly acid taste, and much eaten either raw of pickled. The fruits of *Antidesma acuminatum* Wall. are edible

The leaves of *Antidesma bunius* Spreng. are used as an antidote to snake poison and when young, boiled and used syphilitic cachexia. The bark is considered poisonous, and said to contain an alkaloid.

The bark of *Antidesma ghaesembilla* Gaertn. is considered tonic and astringent, and wood useful as emmenagogue.

The leaves of *Antidesma bunius* Spreng. syn. *A. thwaitesianum* Muell.-Arg. are useful in rheumatism.

The leaves of *Antidesma acidum* Fletz. syn. *A.diandrum* Roth. are used in bile complaints. The whole plant or its part like leaves and fruits are considered useful in blood dysentery. Plant is considered useful in anasarca, bite of rabid dog and jackal, carbuncle, dropsy, muscular pain, pleurisy, pneumonia, sore, dropsy and whitllow. Leaves and fruits are useful in veneral diseases. The fruits are acid and commonly eaten. Leaves are acid and also used as vegetables and in preparing pickles and fruits are also cooked as eatables.

3. KṢETRIKĀ-NASYAHITĀ-NATODARABĪJĀ-ĀDHĀRAŚĀKHĪ-NAGAṆYAVṚNTĀ

A.3 Antirrhinum oronticum Linn.

Scrophiariaceae

Corn Snapdragon.

Erect hreb, 6-18 in. high. Stem much branched from the base, more or less glandular-hairy above. Leaves 1-2 in. long, sub sessile, linear or oblong-lanceolate, entire. Flowers half in. ling, pale-pink streaked with purple. sepals narrow, spreading, longer than the corolla. Capsule 1/3 in. long, pubescent. seeds compressed, concave on one face, back keeled, margins thickened.

Cold season; December to May.

Punjab plains, Salt Range and Qestern Himalayas up to 6,000 ft. North Africa, Europe and the Canaries. Common within the area of Upper Gangetic Plains and Siwalik range; mostly common in the corn fields and cultivated grounds of various localities in regions.

3.1 *Antirrhinum oronticum Linn.* An erect-ascending, simple or much-branched, glandular-hairy, annual herbs. stems often branched from.. the base, glabrous downwards, glandular hairy upwards. Leaves sessile, linear, with a narrowed base, obtuse or subacute, glabrous, 1-6 × 0.1-0.3 cm., with a revolute margin. Flowers in lax, leafy, spiciform racemes. Bracts foliaceous. Pedicels 0.2-0.5 cm. long. Calyx 0.8-1.5 cm long, hairy. Corolla white, purplish-streaked. Capsule obliquely, ovoid, hairy, ± cm. long.

Siwalik range, Uttar Pradesh. Common in grassy lacalities, fields, roadsides, gardens and waste places.

3.2 *Antirrhinum majus Linn.*

Scrophulariacease

Erect, simple or branched, annual-perennial herbs. stems terete, glabreus downwards, gland-hairy upwards. Leaves sessile or short-petioled, ovate-eiiptic to oblong, narrowed towards both ends, glandular. Flowers in many flowered. glandular-hairy, recemes. pedicels 0.5-1 cm. long, glandular-hairy. Calyx 0.5-0.8 cm. long glandular-hairy. corolla white or red or variegated, glandular-hairy outside. with 2 lines of hairs indside the lower lip, 3-6 cm. long. lobes glabrous.

Siwalik range, U.P. Plant cultivated in gardens as an ornamental; often must with as an escape in maste places.March to May. Southern Europe, Syria and North, Africa.

March to May

Native to Southern Europe, Syria and North Africa

3.3 *Schweinfurthia sphaerocarpa A. Br.*

Antirrhinum glaucum Stocks ex Wight.

Screphulariaceae

Sanipat, nepalnimb (Hindi), Senpat (Bombay), Sunpat.

Peremnial, branches 4-12 in. Leaves .5-1.5 in, obtuse or subacute, marrowed into the short petiole. sepals .5 in long, equalling the corolla-tubes, enlarged in fruit. corolla-dirty white. Filaments hairy at the base. capsule 1/4 - 1/3 um diam. seeds pale.

Scinds, in rocky places. Rajputana Desert, Sind, and saluchistan. and Afghanistan.

3.4 Two species of *Antirrhinum linn.* are distinguishable. Leaves linear, calyx-lobes linear, feliaceous, corolla 0.8-1 cm. long and seeds cup-shaped are differential characters in *Antirrhinum erentium* Linn.; whereas *Antirrhinum majus* Linn. is with leaves evate-lanceelate to obleng, calyx-lobes ovate-rounded, not foliaceous, corolla 3-4 cm. long and seeds not cup-shaped.

3.5 Other species of *Schweinfurthia syn. Antirrhinum* is already refered *Schweinfurthia papillionacea* (L.) Boibb. *Antirrhinum papillionaceum* L. *Schweinfurthia Sphaerocarpa* (Banth) A. Braun ex monts.

3.6 The species of *Antirrhinum* Linn. are medicinally useful. The fruits and leaves of *Antirrhinum glaucum* S. ex W. syn. *Schweinfurthia sphaerocarpa* A. Br. are together powdered with stems and recommended in typhoid conditions, powdered plant is snuffed up for bleeding from nose or in epitaxis. The seeds are 'sunpat' of drugists.

Plant drug contains alkaloids.

4. KĀṢṬHAMUḶĀ-GHAṆṬĀPHALĀ-TRIKOṆABĪJĀ-DĪRĞHAŚĀKHĪ-SANDHĀNIKĀ

B4. Byttneria herbacea Roxb.

Sterculiaceae

Adhiubel (Gujarat-Surastra-Kathiwarha), Bekusindur (Santhal); Bir-sindur, Masvasi, Sambarkhai, Sarpapired.

Branched herb with perennial woody root-stock; branches long, slender, sometimes more than a meter long, sub-woody towards the base, 123 mm. in diam, often resting on ground or on neighbouring plants, minutely pubscent, elder branches with black data on one side. Leaves 5-10 cm. long, alternate, often-distant. ovate to narrowly evate or lanceolate, acuminate, unequally toothed, subcordate and trinerved at base; petiole 0.8-1.2 cm. long, slender, pubescent. peduncle very narrow.

1-2 cm. long, axillary or extra-axillary. Capsule pendulous, 0.6-1 cm. acress, pale green covered with short dark green with soft spines, glabrous, 4-5 lobed, dehescent. seeds pale brown, elliptic, bluntly triangular.

August to September, December to January.

Uttar Prdesh, Bihar, North Circars, Deccan, Karnataka and Orissa. Eastern India. Upper Gangetic Plains, Central India, also northern India.

Byttneria herbacea Roxb.

4.1 Creeping fruticose herbs with ascending branches. Leaves up to 2.2 × 1.5 cm., ovate, acuminate, cordate at base, usually with a linear gland at base on lower side of midrib, glabrescent; stipules linear. Flower marroon with yellow anthers.

Central and Southern India; also in Karnataka (dry sandy-rocky terrain the eastern plains). Konkan, Bombay, Madras State (Tamilnadu), Deccan and Car natic.

4.2 B. **Byttneria grandiflora. DC.**

Buetineria aspera Colebr.

Byttneria aspera Colebr. ex Wall ('Buettneria')

Sterculiaceae

Barauk-Pan

Powerful woody climber, often with a trees-like stem. Leaves cordate, entire, glabrous and shining above, blade 5-8, petiole 2-5 in. Capsule globose, 1.5-2 in. diam., armed with many long sharp spines.

May to June.

Sikkim, ascending to 4,000 ft., Khasi Hills, Andamans, Burma,Cochin-China, China.

4.3 Byttneria pilosa Roxb.

Sterculiaceae

Dim-sob-doukha, Dom-shok--doukha

(Cachar hills), Manlang-rang (Kuki),

Jirmi(Khasi); Champhat.

Large woody climber; branchlets grooved, at first densely pubescent, afterwards more or less strigose. Leaves 4-7 by 2-2.5in., orbicular or ovate, cordate, abruptly acuminate, often more or less distinctly, 3-5 lobed, closely serrulose-denticulate membraneous, somethat harshly stellate-pubescent, 7-9 nerved at the base and with 1.5 lateral nerves on either side of the midrib, other nerves as in the precceding species (B. aspera); petiole 2-8 in. long shaggy while young. Flowers yellowish, about .2 in. across; in much branched pubescent compound cymes; brateoles subulate, pedicels capillary several together on utlimate cymose unbels; petals shorter than the sepals, terminal lobe linear lanceolate; anthers yellow, spreading. Capsules spherical, -5-.8 in. diam., densely covered with barbed bristles.

October to January.

Assam prevince; Lower hills; from the foot of Sibsagar hills, Nowgong and other areas in the region.

4.4 Two other species of Byttneria Linn. occurring in India and adjacent regions including Burma, may be indicated;

Buettneria creanulaia Wall. Pegu, Tenasserim. Leaves ovate acuminate, blade 3-4, petiele 1-3 in. long; capsules up to i in. diam., prickles 1/4 in. long.

Buettneria andamanensis Kurz. Andamans, Tenasserim. Leaves 3-5 lobed, capsules 1 in. duam, prickles on a conical base, unequal in length.

4.5 Two species of Buetineria Linn. are distinguishable. Leaves charataceous, entire, glabrate and shining above, and capsule armed with stout conical prickles in Buetineria aspera Colebr.; whereas Buettneria pilesa Roxb. is with membranous and serrulote leaves. more or less pilose above, and capsule and wiry thin barbed bristles. In another species of Bytineria Leefling (Buettneria), the leaves ovate, acuminate, cordate at base, usually with a linear gland at base on lower side of midrib, and capsules 4-5 lobed, dehescent, pale green covered with short dark green soft spines, and other characteristcs.

4.6 Buettneria aspera Colebr.

Sterculiaceae

Tikeuni-borua (Assamese-Sibsagar), Risul-rubi (Miri & Aber.), Warpekhu (Mikyang), Pira-deujha (Kachar Hills), Jong-Bong-rhui (Lushal); Lata-Kuti, Dusi-phri (Gare), Ther-um, Tile-saphei, Mei-Kleng, Mei-Shah (Khasi Hills).

Large woody climber with sulcate branches; young shoots and inflorescence grey or buff stellate pubescent. Bark dark-brown closely longiiudinally or spirally, furrowed on old stems. Leaves 4-8 in. diam., orbicular, cordate, abruptly acuminate, entire or or obscurely repand, charatmeus, glabrate and shining above, puberulous, along the nerves beneath., bright pink, when young; midrib with one or more large glands near the 5-7 nerves base; abd 5-6 regularly arched lateral nerves; tetiaries sub-parallel and transverse to the secondary nerves; ultimate nervules very fine and closely reticulate; petiole 2-5 in. long, sulcate, puberulous; stpules .5 in. long, linear lanceolate, early deciduous. Flowers pale brown, 14-2 in. diam., buds ovoid or pyramidal; pedicels slender, .3-.5 in. long jointed in the middle, cymosely umbelled on the ultimate ramifications of peduncled cymes; inflorescence up to 3 in. long; peduncles fascicled, axillary up to 2 in. long; bracts and bracteoles subulate. Petals shorter than the sepals, terminal lobe fleshy, acute labceolate. Capsules 1-1.5 in. across, globose, woody, armed with stout sharp rather distant conical prickles. seeds evate oblong, selitary in each cell, immersed in watery sap, unarmed.

May to June; November to March.

Assam prvince; fairly common in mixed evergreen forests through-out Upper Assam and Naga hills ascending up to 2,500 ft.

4.7 **Buettneria pilosa** Rexb.

Sterculiaceae

Large climber, the stem as thich as man's thing. Leaves cordate serrulate, shortly, 3-5 lobed, lobes acuminate, blade 5-6, petiole 4-5 in. Capsules globose, 3/4 in. diam., densely covered with long brown rigid but flexible bristles.

May to july.

Eastern Himalayan region; Sikkim up to 4,000 ft.; Assam, Khasi Hills, Manipur, Chittagong, Burma.

4.8 Various species of Byttneria Leefling (Buettneria Linn.) are mediçinally useful. They are also utilised for allied purposes such as herbal detergent and veterinary drugs. The young parts and bark of the plant Buettneria aspera Colebr. are macerated and useful for washing the hairs by women in certain tribal regions.

The rootstock of Buettneria herbacea Roxb. are ground and rubbed an swellings of legs and limbs. It is used in female diseases 'pardhal' (known in Santhals community of tribals).

The bark of plant Byttneria grandiflora DC. syn. B. aspera wall. is used as herbal detergent for washing the hairs by women and folks in some areas of plants availability.

The roots, stem and other parts of plant Byttneria herbacea Roxb. are useful in bone fracture cases. Generally the bark is pounded and pasted over the fractured lesion of body part and properly bandazed with usual measures needed in particular condition or stage.

The stems are ground and applied externally over the body parts swetlings. legs, Upper or lower limbs and other organs affected with oedema including sprains and boils.

The roots are made into paste after grinding well and topically pasted over wounds, ulcers and other similar complaints. including cuts and sores.

Plant is useful in cholera, syphilis, cough, dysentery and stomach troubles. It is used in menorrhagia in females.

The plant is useful as veterinary medicine.

The roots of Byttneria pilosa Roxb. are pounded and applied to sores in cattles as useful herbal measure in veterinary medicine for similar ailments.

5. TIKTAPARṆĪ-KṚMIGHĀTINĪ-ADHOŚĀKHĪ-SUPUṢPĀ-MSṆḌURASUNGĀ

C5. Calycopteris floribunda Lamk.

Calycopteris nutans Kurz.

Getonia floribunda Roxb.

Combretaceae

Ukshi (Marathi). Kyut-ne-nway (Burmese), Khoaray (Hindi). Minnargedi (Tamil). Adivijama (Telugu),

Large scandent shrub, branches drooping, young shoots rusty villous. Leaves opposite, ovate, shortly acuminate, entire. Flowers bisexual, in tomentose terminal and axillary panicles. Free portion of calyx infundibuliform, petals o, stemens 10, inserted in two lines on the inside of the calyx-tube, the 5 upper alternating with the calyx-teeth. Fruit 5-ribbed, villous, in. long, surmounded by the enlarged calyx, the segments of which are 1/2 - 1 in. long.

January to April or May and other months.

Western peninsula, in decidueus forests, Assam. Chittagong, Uppar and Lower Burma.

Western peninsula, in deciduous forests, Assam. Chittagong, Uppar and Lower Burma.

5.1 Calycopteris floribunda (Roxb.) poiret.

Straggling shrubs. Young parts tomentose. Leaves ovate, acuminate. ronnded at base, up to 10 x 5 cm. Calyx white, showy. Fruit short brownish, yellow-tomentose.

Indo-malaysia. Common in undergrowth of lower ghats, Karnataka state, southern India.5.2 The plant Calycopteris floribunda Lamk. is medicinally useful, and various parts are used as medicine.

The leaves are bitter, astringent, anthelmintic, laxative and antispasmodic.

Leaves are used in colic. leaves are ground and administered with butter as cure of dysentery and malaria; Leaves are also used as external application to ulcers and wounds.

Roots are considred antidote to snaks bite.

Plant contains calyccopterin; and leaves centain 7%, tannin. Leaves yield 0.28-0, 29% calyocopterin. Calyocopterin more toxic to earthworms than santonin or oil of chenepodium but less toxic than thymol.

Leaves are applied over cuts and bruises. Leaves are considered useful for application to white patches on skin externally, and they are internally given in worms camplaints.

6. KAṆṬAKṢUPĀ-TŪLADHARĀ-BALYĀ-KṚṢIBHŪMIJĀ-VĀMIKĀ

Cirsium argyracanthus DC.

Cnicus argyracanthus (DC.) Clarke. (excl var.)

Asteraceae

Erect robust herb, 1-2 m. high, with rough or cottony stem. Leaves alternate, sessile, irregularly pinnately lebed, margins best with lone rigid spines, glabrous, or cottony beneath, radical leaves stalked and larger. Heads discoid, 2-2.5 cm. acroos, sessile or shortly stalked, crowded in terminal and and axillary clusters. Outer involucral bracts, ending in long rigid spines, innermost linear, long-pointed. Flowers pale-yellow or white. Pappus feathery, united at base.

May to September.

Temperate Himalayas from Pakistan to Bhutan. Siwaliks in Uttar Pradesh (Dehradun), in damp waste places.

6.1 Cirsium wallichii DC. Var. fasciculatum (Hook. F.) Raizada. syn. Cnicus wallichii (DC.) Hk. f. var. fasciculata MK.f.

Breea arvensis (L.) Less. syn. Cirsium arvensis (L.) scop. Cirsium involucratum DC.

Cirsium verulum (Don.) Spr.

The plants of Cirsium wallichii DC. (from Siwaliks, Dehradun) are referable to var. fasciculatum (hook. f.) Cnicus wallichii var. fasciculata Hook. g. Since the species is very variable in habit, shape and size of leaves, hairiness, shape and size of involucral bracts, and nature of the inflorescence the characters on which varieties in J.D. Hooker Flora are based, the taxon together with other five varieties recognised (Hook. f.) are to be examined thoroughly before treating them as distinct vaieties.

6.2 Cnicus wallichii Hook. f. var. fasciculata Hook. F. is very spinous; and leaves white-tomentose or cottony beneath; heads fascicled; inner invol-bracts with long lanceolate dilated spinescent tips. Siwaliks and foot hills, Uttar Pradesh.

Cirsium chinensis Card et Chap. and Cirsium involucratun DC. also occur in Khasi hills, Assam.

6.3 Cirsium arvense (Linn.) Scop.

Serratula arvensts Linn.

Cnicus arvensis (Linn.) Hoffm.

***Cardus lanatus* Roxb.**

Asteraceae (Compositae).

Erect, thistle-like herbs, with subterranean sotolons. Stems erect, simple or branched, cottony. Leaves sessile, pinnatilobed-fid to-partite, prominently nerved, glabrescent or cottony above, white-lanate or-woolly beneath; segments acicularly dentate, 4-7 (-10) cm. long. Heads solitary, 1.5-2 cm. acress, subsessile or on a short peduncle. Involucral bracts 4 to 5-seriate; outer ones ovate, shortly aciculate, cottony. 0.5 cm. long; inner ones lanceolate, glabrous, with acicular, dilated, recurved tips, 1 cm. long. Flowers 1.8-2 cm. long, with purple corollas. Corolla-lobes 0.4-9.5 cm. long. Achenes oblong, glabrous, with a truncate apex. Pappus-hairs plumose, dirty white er brownish white, connate at base, deciduous, Receptacle flat, with filiform, bristly pales.

February to May or June.

Plains of Bengal and Punjab, Western Himalayas from Kum'ason to Kashmir, ascending to 12.000 ft. in Western Tibet; also in China and from West and North Asia to Europe.

6.4 *Cnicus arvensis* Heffm.

Erect leafy horb. Stems many from the perennial creeping root, 2-3 ft. high, not winged, usually simple, cobwebby tementose above, the sexes forming separate tufts. Leaves sessile, 3-5 in. long, linear-oblong or obovate, sinuate or pinnatifid, scabrid above, .white tomentose or woolly beneath; lobes divergent, tipped with spines. Heads dioecious, solitary fascicled or corymbose, those of the males globose, 1/2-1 in. in diam; the female heads much longer and with more lax involucral bracts. Involucral bracts glabrate or cobewebby; outer most short, ovate or triangular-ovate, ending in a short spine; inner gradually. longer, with undulate often recurved tips; innermost linear lanceolate, scarious. Corolla dull purple, its limb, 5-partite. Achenes smooth, shining. Pappus light brown.

Abundant weed within the areas of Upper Gangetic Plains, Sub-Himalayan tracts, Siwaliks and adjacent regions; especially on cultivated grounds agricultural fields and watercourses.

6.5 Cirsium lepskyle Pteral.

Cnicus griffthii Hook. f.

Asteracese

Soh-Chiia (Khasi), Sumori-Kaura (Nepali).

Thistle-like herb. Leaves sessile or base auricled, 2.5-6 in. by 7-2.5 in., pinnatifid; lobes lanceolate, acute, spinescent, setulose above, white tomentose beneath. Heads bisexual Involucral-bracts many seriate; outer short with acicular apex, the rest linear-wavy, asistate or acuminate. Corolla 1.25 in. long, 5-lobed. Anther-base sagitate, auticled, tails slender. Style-arms short, obtuse. Cypsela obevoid-oblong, obtusely 4-angled. Pappus copious, feathery, unequal, up to 1 in. long the longer hairs ususlly clavellate.

Cold season.

Assan state, Khasi hills, ascending up·to 6,000 ft. Mishmi hills, Uppar Assam.

6.6 *Crisium wallichii* DC

Asteraceae

Errct, annual-perennial, thistle-like herbs. Stems robust, simple or branched, ribbed, glabrescent or cottony. Basal leaves pinnatifid-partite or 2-pinnate; upper ones lanceolate, pinnatilobed-fid, glabrescent or cottony on the upper surface, white-lanate or wooly on the lower surface; segments acicularly lobed or dentate. Heads 2-4 cm. across, terrminal, sessile or on short peduncles, in dense fascicles. Outer involucral bracts ovate, cottony, aciculate; inner ones lanceolate, with aciculate, dilated tips. 1-1.5 cm. long. Corolla 1.5 cm. long Pappus-hairs dirty white or brown.

February to August.

Common Himalayan species and occurs also on the Nilgiri hills.

6.7 Various species of Cirsium Linn. are medicinally useful and also used in other purposes.

The plants of Cirsium arvense (Linn.) Scop. are emetic, tonic and diaphoretic.

Plant centains glucoside, essential oil, alkaloid. Seeds contain 21.9% fatty oil; and plant contains a volatile alkaloid and essential, and onicin, a crystaline bitter glycoside, possessing emetic and emmanogogue properties.

The roots of the plant Cirsium sinensis C. B. Glarke syn. Cnicus sinensis Gardner & Champ. are used internally for flatulence and externally for ulcers and abscesses.

The stems and leaves of plant are antiscorbutic.

The seeds of Cirsium involucratum DC. are edible. The young shoots are vegetative. Plant is called Sen-Chila.

The seeds of Cirsium lepskyle Petr. are edible, and the leaves and young sheets are used as vegetable.

The roots of Cirsium verulum (Den.) Spr. are useful for their cooling properties. Plant is useful as diaphoretic. Roots are used as expectorant. Roots are considered tonic and useful in general debility.

Leaves of plant are applied to wounds and ulcers.

Plant is also of veterinary medicine uses. Leaves are useful as galactagogue.

The stems of *Cirsium wallichii* DC. are edible.

The roots of plant Breea arvensis (L.) Less. syn. *Cirsium arvensis* (L.) Scop. are useful as diuretic medicine.

7. RASAPŪRṆĀŚAKAKAKṢUPĀ-PĪTAPUPṢPĀ RODHĀSRIKĀ-BĀLUJĀ

Crassocephalum crepidioides (Bth.) Moore.

Gynura crepidioides Benth.

Erechtites valerianifolia Senus Fiseher; (non (Wolf DC)

Asteraceae (Cempesitae)

Akatasu, Gendahamang, Jati, Sagon-nadi

Erect succulent usually much branched annual herb about 33-52 em. high. stem and branches pubescent or nearly glabrous. Leaves alternate, spathulate, usually, deeply lyrate-pinnatifid, sometimes not lobed. mostly petiolate, the upper ones rearly sessile, 2.5-15 cm. long; on long slender pedicels, in a dense or lax corymbose cyme, rarely solitary. Disk hairy with filiform bracts below. Involucral bracts about 15, linear-subulate, glabrous or slightly stutulose. Florets all tubular, hermophrodite or rarely a few outer ones female; limb 5-toothed. Corolla orange-yellow, or tinged with purple, shorter than or equalling the pappus. style branches slender, tips long, subulate, hispid. Anther-bases entire or subauricled. Achenes narrow, many ribbed. Pappus hairs copious, fine, white.

Cold season; October to May.

Native of tropical Africa. Found all over Assam, Bengal, Madhya Pradesh (Bastar), Kalahande state in Orissa. Burma. Uttar Pradesh (Dehradun).

7.1 Crasssocepheum crepidioides (Bentham.) S, Moore.

Slender, erect herbs. Leaves 15 x 4 cm. elliptic-lanceolate, acute-acuminate, narrowed below, somewhat lobed, glabrous. Florets red.

Africa, now Pantropical. Common in plains and Ghats along roadsides outskirts of forests and on sandy river beds.

7.2 The plants of *Crassocephalum crepidioides* (Bth.) Moore are mediciually useful.

Leaves are useful in constipation. Leaves are applied to cuts, injuries as haemostatic remedy. leaves are also useful in headache. Leaves are considered useful in stomach disturbance. Plant is edible and leaves are used as vegetable. Leaves are fish bait.

8. MEGHANĪLA-MṚGAPADĪ-VṚNTIKĀ-NAG-NAPUṢPADHARĀ-SUNETRĀ

E8.

Emilia sonchifolia (L.) DC.

Cacalia sonchifolia Linn.

Asteraceae (Compositae)

Hirankhuri (Hindi), Sahimodi, Sudhimudi (Bengla),

Sadamandi (Bombay), Mulshevi (Malayalam); Dodigaru, Neethi-dodi.

Erect, often muticauline, annual-perennial, somewhat glausecent herbs. Stems branched at base, often decumbent ascending, glabrous or so. Leaves sessile; lower ones often resolute, narrowed to the base, with an entire-dentate lower part, passing into ovate-triangular, orbicular or reniform, dentate upper part, 5-15 cm. long; upper ones sagitate, acute, dentate, with rounded basal auricles, glabrescent or so. Heads ¯cm. long, on 2.5-5 cm. long peduncles, combined into corymbs. Involucral bracts 8-10, lanceelate, acute, 0.6-0.7 cm. long, shorter than the florets. Corolla purple or reddish purple, 0.9-1 cm. long. Achenes with 5 hairy ribs alternating with faint, glabrous ribs, 0.3-0.4 cm. long. Pappus-hairs white, ¯0.6 cm. long.

January to December; greater part of the year; August-September Throughout-India, ascending to 5,000 ft. in the Himalayas. Ceylon, China and tropical and subtropical Africa, and in America (introduced).

8.1 *Emilia sonchifolia* DC.

Slender semewhat glaucous herb, 10-18 in. high, glabrous puberulous or scabrid. stems erect, or diffuse and often rooting at the nedes, more or less branched. Leaves 1.5 to 4 in. long; lower petioled, lyrate-pinnatified or obovate, entire or sinuate; upper smaller, amplexcaul, with acute or obtuse auricles. Heads half inch long. solitary or laxly corymbose; peduncles very slender, nodding when young. involbracts nearly equalling the flowers. linear-oblong, acute, narrowly margined. corollas pinkish-violet or white. stylearms semi-cylindric, the tip conic. Achenes small, with 5-ribbed scabrid.

Upper Gangetic plains, Sub-Himalayan tracts and Siwaliks; common within the area, occurring commonly specially in shady, humid, localities, agricultural fields, farms, gardens, forest edges, ravine boarders and other similar areas.

8.2 Emilia sonchifolia DC. An erect, glauceus herb. Leaves crenate. us to 10 × 4 cm.; well-developed lower leaves lyrate or with narrow base and triangular to orbicular terminal segments; upper leaves lanceolate, semiamplexicaul. Involucral bracts or involucre 7-9 × 2-3 mm., equalling the florets. corolla lobes 0.5-0.7 mm. long.

Pantropical; Asia and Africa. Southern India, common in Ghats, often weeds in estates and disturbed areas, Karnataka.

8.3 Emilia sonchifolia DC. Erect or diffuse, scabrid or puberulous glabrous herb. Radical leaves spreading, usually stalked, more or less pinnatified, lobed entire or coarsely toothed, terminal lobe much the largest. Stem. leaves few, alternate, similar to the radical or lanceolate or ovate, stem clappping or base lobed. Heads discoid, long-stalked, corymbose. Involcres in one series, narrow, equal, edges often copious or edges often more or less united, reflexed in fruit; receptacles flat, naked. Flowers purple, pappus white and copious and achenes with bristly angles.

Northern India; Himachal Pradesh, valleys below Simla; Uattar Pradesh hills; ascending in the Himalayan reginen up to 2,000m. elevattion.

8.4 Emilia sonchifolia DC. A slender nearly glabrous herb up to about 20 ft. high, with lanceolate upper caulie leaves or oblong-lanceolate, auricled, lower leaves 2-4 in. long; heads small, few-flowered; involucres connate, tubular splitting into 8-10 segments in fruit; receptacles naked; corolla lobe short, resy; cyssela 5-angled and white papus, soft. Eastern Himalaya and eastern region; Assam province, Khasi hills, ascending to 4,000 ft. elevation.

8.5 Emilia prenanthoidea DC.

Emilia angustifolia DC.

Cocalia angustifolia Wall.

Erect, glabrous, rarely scabrid, slender herb. Lowest leaves small ovate petioled or 0, all or upper sessile, linear oblong obtuse or acute nearly entire deeply sagitately or breadly auricled at the base. Involucres shorter than the scarlet flowers, style arms dilated at the tip; achenes glabrous.

Eastern Himalayas; Sikkim Himalayan region and Khasia mountains, 2.000-4,000 sf. elevations, upper Burma.

8.6 Emilia flammea Cass.

Emilia sonchifolia var. sagitata Clarke.

Cocalia- mucronate Heyne.

C. coccinea

Emilia sagitata DC.

Asteracese

Erect, glabrous, or scabrid herb. Lower leaves petioled obovate or subspathulate entire or toothed, upper large oblong or ovate-oblong deeply sagitately auricled. Involucral bracts much shorter than the scarlet flowers. Achenes 5-ribbed scabrid. Style-arms semi-cylindric tip conic.

Konkan, India. Native of China, natiralised in India. Philippines Islands. Also cultivated in gardens.

8.7 Emilia javanica (Burn. F.) C.B. Robinsen

Emilia sagitata DC.

E. flammes Cass

Hieracium javanicum Burm. f.

Erect glabrous or scabrid herb; lower leaves petiled, obevate or subspathulate, entire or toothed; upper leaves large, oblong or evate-oblong, deeply sagitately auricled. Involures much shorter than the flowers; achenes 5-ribbed, scabrid, style-arms half-cylndric and tip cenical. Concan (Konkon), Southern states, Khasi Hills in India.China, Japana, Siam (Thailand), Philippines, Tropical Africa and other regions.

8.8 Emilia alstonii Foeberg.

Asteraceae

Short stemmed with ascending inflorescences. Leaves crenate, up to 4 × 2 cm., longer ones becoming pinnatifid with ovate terminal segments, the upper becoming lanceolate to bract-like. Involucre ca. 8 x 4 mm. Corolls purplish, exerted about one quarter in length; lebes 1.4-1.5 dm. long. Anthers 0.6-0.8 mm. long.

Sri Lanka, tresturn Karnataka, Common used in wet deciducous to evergreen forests, Karnataka State.

8.9 Emilia exserta Fosb.

Asteraceae

Stems diffuse, coarsely branched herbs. Leaves up to 3 × 9.5 mm., shallowly crenate to dentate, the lower ones with a reniform terminal segments and narrow to broadly winged petiole sometimes winged petiole beomes lyrate), upper leaves lancoslate with truncate to semiamplexicaul base. Involucre 6.7 × 5 mm. Corolla purple, exserted about one-third its length, lobes 2.0-2.3 mm long.

Sri Lanka, Western Karnataka. Common in partial to full sun semi-evergreeen to wet deciduous forests, Karnataka Etate.

8.10 Plants of *Emilia sonchifolia* (Linn.) DC. are ver variable, in habit, hairiness, and the size, shape and lobation of leaves. in different areas of occurrence as taxa show much variation in field.

There species of *Emilia* Cass. are distinguishable by floral characters, habit and other features with difference. Corolla lobes to 0.7 mm. long. (less than 1 mm) is in *Emilia sonchifolia* (L.) DC; whereas length exceeds in other species. Corolla lobes over i mm. long in two species which are separated by other characters. Corolla lobes ca. 1.5 mm. long, anthers ca. 6.7 mm. long in small plants, densely branched with short stems in *Emilia alstonii* Fosberg; when *Emilia exserta* Fesb. is with corolla lobes cs. 2 mm. long, antthers ca. 1.2 mm. long in large plants basely branched, with elongate stems.

8.11 Emilia alstonii Fesb. is semetimes considered intermediate with E. exsera Fesb., and probably E. exserta intermediate with the former. There seems to stronger tendency for the basal leaves to have more reniform terminal segments as in case of E. alstenii it can be with a different aspect and and anthers 1.0 mm. long, and *E. exerta* similarly much more dentate than others from varietally different plants. Quite variable weed *Emilia sonchifolia* DC (earlier with three or more varieties) is closely allied to *Emilia flammes* cass which sometimes approaches the larger form of *E. sonchifolia*, but the lower leaves seem to be always entire and the scarlet heads broader. *Emilia prenanthoidea* DC. very slender species with much the habit of *E. flammes,* but with few or radical leaves, and with glabrous achenes. *E. zeylanica* Clarke very closely resembles *E. prenanthoides* in all but the achenes and style-arms *E. walkeri* Hook. f. is a much larger plant than any of the preceeding species, with specific features, and synonymous to *E. prenanthoidea* Tawaites.

8.12 Emilia javanica (Burm. F.) C.B. Robinson and *E. sagitata* DC. are sometimes considered as two distinct species, and their hardly any specific distinction find them as one polymorphic species.

These taxa have significance of biological aspect of the characters and their role in the evolution of an the relationship of the elder as well as newer taxa naming with in binomials species alongwith biosystematics for presence of ecotypes and cytotypes, and polymorphism in case of various taxa accounted fao *Emilia* **Cass.** which is taxonomically interesting.

8.13 The sepcies of *Emilia* cass. are medicinally useful. Plant *Emilia sagitata* DC. syn. *E. flammes* Cass. is considered useful in children ailments.

The decoction of whole plant of *Emilia sonchifolia* DC. is used as a febrifuge, in fevers of children. The decoction is useful in infantile tympanitis and in bowel complaints.

The juice of leaves of the plant is useful in eyes inflamation, night blindness and sore eyes, and also in allied eye ailments.

The roots of plant are considred useful in diarrhoea and similar bowel troubles.

Leaves are pounded and applied over wounds and ulcers. They are externally applied over inflammation in affected parts. Leaves are used for bruises and cuts topically. Whole plant and leaves are considred to have cooling properties and useful in burning sensation of whole body and either allied complaints. Leaves are useful for their cooling effect in the form of fusion or powder. They are also externally applicable.

The roots and leaves are considered useful in eyes diseases specially catract and other common complaints.

Leaves and roots are ground and applied to foul sores, chronical wounds and gangrenes.

Plant is also edible particularly leaves which are found useful as salad or any other form including vegetable.

9. HARITAVALLĪ-PĪTAKUSUMĀ-KRṢNAPHALĀ-GHANAROMAKIṬṬĀ-MUKHAPRIYĀ

Erycibe paniculata Roxb.

Erycibe paniculata var. **wightiana** (Grah.) Cl.

Convolvulaceae

Ankote (Kannada), Unankodi (Tamil), Kari (Santhal), Niguniboal-lota (Assam), Puttapaliga (Telugu), Trimptyatali (Malayalam); Baralekeshar, Kari.

Large climbing evergreen shrub, or occasionally a small erect tree; branches long, more or less angular, clothed when young with reddish-brown, tomentose. Leaves 3-5 in. long, elliptic-oblong or obovate-oblong, abruptly acuminate, narrowed towards the base into a short petiole glbrous or nearly so; main lateral nerves 4-6 pairs, arcuate. Flowers yellow in long terminal or occasionally axillary panicles, densely rusty-tementose. Calyx clothed outside with reddish-brown tomentum and more or less stallate-pubescent. Sepals orbicular. Corolls tube broadly funnel-shaped; lobes 5, bifid, hairy on the back below the division, marigins plicate, Anthers with along curved apiculate connective. Bearry subglobose or elipsoid, supported on the persistent calyx, black and pulpy when ripe.

May to November, February to April, Octobber-March.

Regions from Nepal eastwards ascending to 4,000 ft. on Himalaya, and from Bengal and Central province to southern India, and Ceylon, extending to Burma, the Malay Islands and the Malaya Archipelago and Australia.

9.1 Erycibe paniculata Roxb.

Large evergreen woody climber; with bark grey thin, blaze cream coloured, and wood with floral design, phloem pale when first expressed, soon turning deep dirty brown. Leaves 3.5-5 by 1.2-2.2 in., ovate-oblong, abruptly acuminate, entire, coriacecus, glabrous, bark glossy green above when mature, pale beneath; lateral nerves 4-6 on either half, arcuate; base acute; petiole. 3-6 cm. long. Flowers fragrant, yellowish in usually terminal rusty tomentose, panicled drooping cymes up to 7 in. long; pedicels.2 in.

long; calyx ferruginous-tomentose; corolla campanulate; lobes marginate, crisped; stamens included; filaments dilated at the base; anthers with a curved crown; stigmas sessile, sub-globose, often 3-lobed. Berry ellipsoids .3-5. in. in diam., black when ripe, pulp dark purple. Seeds elliptic. Assam province, Lakhimpur, Darnang and Sibsagar. Bengal and eastern region.

9.2 Erycibe paniculata Roxb, Young shoots and inflorescences densely clothed with rust-coloured tomentum. Leaves elliptic-oblong, abruptly acuminate, blade 3-5, petiole 1/3 in. long. flowers yellowish-white, in elongate narrow terminal panicles, petals crisped. Berry about 1/3 in. diam., black when ripe.

Sub-Himalayan tracts of Uttar Pradesh Terai or Rohilkhand, northern Oudh, eastern U.P. bordering Nepal, also in Bundelkhand, Upper Gangetic Plains, Singhbum. Throughtout the Greater parts of country.

9.3 Erycibe paniculata Roxb. Woody, rusty-tementose climbers. Leaf elliptic-lanceolate, cuspidate, shortly acute at base, 7-10 by 2-4.5 cm., glabrous with age, shining. panicle manyflowered. Sepals suborbicular, up to p.3 cm. long. Corolla pale white, 1 cm. long. Anthers apiculate. Berry black, shining up to 2 x 1 cm.

India including Himalayas and Andaman Islands, Sri Lanka. Occasienal in upper Ghats, Karnataka. Andaman and Nicobar Islands, and Western Peninsula.

9.4 Erycibe subspicata Wall.

Euphorbicasae

Branchlets angular, rusty tomentose. Leaves 2-4 by 1-1.8 in., elliptic-lanceolate or broadly elliptic-acuminate, coriaceeus, glabrous; lateral nerves 4-5 on either half, slender; base obtuse or acute; petiole. 2-3.3 in. long. Flowers large in subspicate rusty-tementose, peduncled cymes; inflorescence narrow, spiciform.

Assam, Kamrup, Guwahati, Khasi hills. Upper Burma and Yuman.

April or around.

9.5 Erycibe glaucescens Wall.

Euphorbiaceae.

Glabrous diffuse or sub-scandent shrub. Leaves 2-3 by .9-1.5 in., elliptic-acuminate, entire, coriaceous, glabrous; lateral nerves

5-6 on either half, rather slender and obscure; base cuneate; petiole .2-3. in. long; cymes.axillary or in terminal panicles. Flowers white, fragrant. Corolla lobes rusty-pubescent on the back, petals with a firm musty-silky back.

September or around.

Assam, Cachar, Sylhet. Tenasserim, Burma.

9.6 Erycibe schimiditti Craib.Erycibe laevigata Wall.

Euphorbiaceae

Large straggling or climbing shrub. Branchlets sparsely pubsecent; older branches dark purplish. Leaves 2.5-6 in., elliptic or oblong-elliptic, acuminate, distantly glandular, denticulate, sinute, coriaceeus, glabrous; lateral nerves numerous; midrib impressed above, stout and prominent beneath, tertiaries distinctly and elongately reticulated; base rounded or cuneate; blade 3-7 petiole .3-5 in. long. Flowers yellowish, or yellowish-white usually in axillary short panicles. Berry globose, .75 in. in diam.

December to February

Eastern Himalayan and north-eastern regions, Sikkim (3-5,000 ft. elevation), Khasi hills, Sibasgar.

9.7 Erycibe albiflora Hallifer f.

Euphorbiaceae

Large climber; seem pale purplish; weed on transverse secition with floral design. Leaves 4-6 by 1.3-2 in., oblong lanceolate, acuminate, entire, ceriaceeus, glabrous; lateral nerves 4-6 on either half, conspicuous, arcuate, making an angle of about 30^0 with the midrib; base cuneate. Flowers pale-white in long terminal ferruginous tomentose panicle. Calyx rusty-tomentose externally. Corolla bi-lobed stigmas conspicuously 5-lobed like a strand. fruit ovoid, .5 .3 in.

November to Ferbruary

Assam, Cachar, N.C. Hills.

9.8 Various species of *Erycibe* Roxb. are distinguishable as they are broadly gruped in view of major characters. The brancholets densely rusty-tomentese and inflorescences terminal and axillary in *Erycibe paniculata* Roxb. and some other species xiz. *Erycibe wightiana* Grah., *E. peguensis* Prain, *E. spicate* wall and *E. expanea* Wall.; whereas the branchlets. are glabrous or nearly so, and inflorescences mostly axillary in the rest of species which are separated by two kinds of characteristics. Tertiary nerves distinct, parallel and reticulate in *Erycibe laevigata* Wall., *E. wallichii Prain ex Wallier, E. griffithii Clarke. and E. wallichii prain ex Wallier, E. griffithii* Clarke. and *E. staptiana prein;* whereas the tetary nerves in distincti, underside of leaves minutely granular in *Erycibe coriacea* Wall. syn. *E. fragrans* Wall. and *E. glaucescens* Wall.

9.9 Some other species of *Erycibe* may be indicated : *Erycibe citriniflora* Griff. *E. glomerata* Wall ex choisy *Erycibe curiacea* wall ex Choisy. *E. fragrans* wall ex G. Don. *E. Coriacea Var. fragrans* (Wall ex G. Davi) cl. *Erycibe peguensis* (Cl) Prain. *E. paniculata* var. *peguensis cl. E. paniculata* non. Roxb. *E tomentosa* Bl. *Erycibe tomentosa* B. *E. princii* Wall ex Choisy.

The plants of *Erycibe paniculata* Roxb. are medicially useful and also utilised in other allied purposes. The fruits (ripening nearly after 12 months) are sweet and eaten as edible varatable item. The bark is given in the condition of cholera.

Plant is considered useful in gums trouble. Bark is useful in syphilis. The plant is recommended as hypotensive drug and useful in cases of hypertension.

Plant has uses in veterinary medicine. The leaves and stems are useful in sprains of cattles.

The fruits are edible.

10. GĀRGUVṚKṢA-HASTPRIYĀ-RANGCARMĀ-VIṢAMAPAKṢIKĀ-MŪTRĀMAYAGHANĪ

G10. *Garuga pinnata* Roxb.

Debadabi (Nepali), Armu (Kol), Titmer (Uttar Pradesh-Kumaon), Karur (South.), Gharri (Gend), Kudak (Marathi), Godda (Kannada), Garuga, Gargu (Telugu), Chinyok (Burmese).

Kharpat, Ghoger (Cudh), Kakad, Tejhi, Timur-araung,

The leaves one foot or more, pubescent, when young, afterwards glabrous; leaflets ovate, obtuseky acuminate, oblique, crenate. Flowers 1/2 – 1/4 in. long, in large compound pubescent panicles. Calyx-teeth ovate. Petals linear, inserted between the calyx-teeth. Disk completely clothing the tube of the calyx. Stamens about equalling the petals. Ovary ovoid, tapering into the hairy style; stigmas capitate, 3-lobed.Drupe black about the size of a gooseberry. Aprril to May and October to November.

Widely distributed throughout India, chiefly in mixed deciduous forests.

10.1 Garuga pinnata Roxb.

Large deciduous tree, young shoots and inflorescence grey pubescent. Leaves imparipinnate, orowded near the ends of branches, leaflets 6-9 pairs, opposite or nearly so, lanceolate or ovate-lanceolate, crenate. Flowers yellow, in axillary panicles, several at the ends of branches. Calyx campanulate, 10-ribbed, 5-cleft, lined by a thick disk with a crenate margin, on the edge of which the 5-petals and 10-stamens are inserted. Ovary 4-5celled, 2 collateral ovules in each cell. Fruit a globose fleshy drupe, enclosing 2, rarely more, bony. 1-seeded, tuberculated stones. Subhimalayan tract and moist valleys, ascending to 5,000 ft. from the Jumna eastwards, often in sal forests. Deciduous forests in the greater part of the western peninsula and Burma.

Leafless during the greater part of the dry season. Fresh leaves or foliage in April or May, with flower or after floweing. Plant grows readily from cuttings. Trees feaquently associated with trees of Odina wodier in the Upper Gangatic peains and Sub-Himalayan or foot hill regions.

10.2 Garuga pinnata Roxb. Decidueus trees, deciduous. Leaflets more than 10; basal ones reduced in size, glabrous with age. Flowers yellow. Calyx pubescent; petals ovate, pubescent. Drupe black, 5-seeded.

India, Burma. occasional in western plains, in and around Mallipatana (Hassan distirct), Karnataka state. Region east ward to Burma, and south to the Nilgiris, ascending to outer Himalayas; Upper Gangetic plains, Siwaliks and Terai and adjacent areas in Uttar Pradesh (Dehradun, Saharanpur, Oudh, Rohilkhand, Goakhpur and other areas)

10.3 Garuga pinnata Roxb. A small or medium-sized deciduouts tree upto 7 ft. girth and 60 ft. High. Bark roughish, dark brown sometimes almost silvery at others blackish in parts, exfoliating in irregular wooly scales. Blaze. 9-1 in., spft, not or very shprtly fibrous, without distinct fibrous hands, pink to reddish-brown. Young shoets pubescent. Leaves alternate. 6-18 in. long, Leaflets 11-21, up to 4 by 1.5 in., ovate or oblong oblong-lanceolate, crenate, long-acuminate, oblique, more or less pubescent on both surfaces even when mature. Petiolules. 1-2 in. long. Flowers .25 in. long, yellow, in axillary tomentose pancles 6-12 in. long appealing with or before the leaves, crowded fowards the ends of the shoots. Drupe .7-1-.2 in. dism., globose, smooth, greeniwh-yellow; containing 1-4 pyrenes.

Plant occurring throuhout the Uttar Pradesh hilly region in Kumaon region up to 3,500 ft. as fairly common in dry miscellanous forests. It flowers in spring or March to April and fruits in autumn or September to October.

10.4 Various parts of plant *Garuga pinnata* Roxb. are medicially useful; and they are utilised in other purposes of economic utility Fruits are stomachic. Juice of leaves mixed with honey given in asthma.

Juice of stem dropped into the eye to cure opacities of the conjunctiva.

The bark is employed for tanning, and a greenish-yellow gum-resin exudes from bark of the plant.

The acid drupe is eaten row, pickled or cooked, and the foliage is valued as fodder for cattles patticularly the elephants.

The leaves are use in asthma add used as astringent in some ailments.

Bark in the form of powder or decoction is useful in the cases of diabetes. Juice is also useful in simlar urinary troubles specially glycosuria.

Fruits are useful in dysentery. Bark is useful in eye diseases. Bark is also grounded and applicable over wounds and ulcens.

Roots are useful in skin diseases and veneral diseases. Fruits are edible and pickled. Bark yields dye of black colour. Bark is also fish poison.

11. RAMIVṚKṢAKA-SAUTRIKĀ-PĪTAPRASAVĀ-BAHUŚĀKHĪ-MĪNASAMMOHIKĀ

G.11. *Gnidia glauca* (Fresen) Gilg.

Lasiosiphon glaucus Freson

Gnidia eriocephala Graham.

Lasiosiphon eriocephalus (Graham) Descaisne.

Thymelaeaceae

Ramita, Rametta, Rami (Marathi), Nac-hinaar (Tamil), Mukute, Enujariaga (Kannada), Nangu, Nanca (Malayalam).

Small tree or large much-branched shrub of about 1.8 to 3.0 metre high, leaves alternate, 4-7 x 0.8-1.4 cm., linear eolong abruptly acute, subcordate. Bracts silky. Calyx tube white-hairy, densely so at base; lobes 5, yellow. Disc annular. Ovary stalked, villous. Flowers small, yellow. Disc annular. Ovary stalked, villous. Flowers small, yellow, in dense terminal globose heads. Fruit ellipsoid-oblong, pointed, enclosed in perianth. Bark grey, rather smooth, inner bark fibrous.

Cold season; January

East Africa, Penisular India, Sri Lanka. Wet dociduus forests, Karnataka state. Western Ghats of Bombay and Madras States (Naharastra and Tamilnaudu) ascending to 7,000 ft. in the Niligiris. Open forests on the hills of Deccan and Western Ghats from Knokan souhwards to Kerala, Nilgiri, Palni and Tinnevelly hills ascending the atitudes of 1200-2.100 metres.

11.1 Gnidia glauca var. **insularia** (Gaertn.) Townseed.

Lasiosiphon eriocephalus sensu Hook. f.

Large shrubs. Endemic to Ceylon.

11.2 Gnidia L. and **Lasiosiphon** Fresen are treated as congeneric.

11.3 The plant *Gnidia eriocephalus* Decne. is medicinally useful, and of economic importance and utility in other purposes.

The bark and leaves of the plant are acrid and piseneus. They are used as fish poisen which is not fatal to fishes but stupefying effect as the fishes, after applying thing plant, do not die but float along the streams in a stunned condition.

The bark contains a vascicant resin.

The plant causes dermatitis. The leaves are applied to swellings and contusiens. The stain bark guilds filre bark is usful for tying bundles and filre pulp is suggested for bleached paper.

12. KṢṬHATARU-PUṢPAGANDHĀ-GRANTHISRUVĀ-RAKTASKNDANĪ-ROMILAKARṆIKĀ

H12. *Hopea odorata* Roxb.

Dipterocarpaceae

Thengan, Thingan (Burmese)

Evergreen, wood yellowish-brown, close-and even-grained, very durable. Glabrous, except infloresence. Leaves ovate-lanceoraṭe, secondary nerves 12 pairs. Flowers fragrant, in axillary grey tomentose, panicles, petals ciliate at margin, anthers oblong. ovary gradually narrowed into conical stylopodium and long cylindrical style. Ovary and stylopodium puberulous.

March to April; May to June.

Moist forests in the southern portion of the Eastern Peninsula, from Pegu and Tenasserim to Cochinchina, Andamans. Also in Chittagong in Bengla Desh. Not gregarious but scattered in mixed forests.

12.1 Hopea punga (Dennst.) Malberly.

Hopea wightiana Wall.

Artocarpus punga Dennst.

Dipterocarpaceae

Kevsi (Marathi), Haiga (Kannada), Ha Pangu (Tamil) Youngest branchesto and petioles seftly, pubescent, otherwise glabrous. Leaves ceriaceous, oblong, 6-8 in. long, petiole short. Flowers in axillary fascicled panicles, shorter than the leaves, petals pubescent outside. Upper portion of ovary puberulous, stylopodium glabrous, slightly verucose, style short. Round echinate galls frequent in the axilla of leaves.

March to June; April to May.

Evergreen forasts at the feet of the Western Ghats from North Kanara seuthwards. Often gregarious, covering large forests in the low country of South Kanara.

12.2 Hopea wightiana Wall. ex Wight.

Evergreen trees up to 20 metres high. leaves up to 24 x 6.5 cm., lanceolate, abruptly acute, subtruncate at base. Sepals glabrous; petals ovate-lanceolate, pubsecent, Stamens 15. Accrescent calyx lobes up to 5 x 2 cm., erect, oblong, reddish. South-West India. Common in semi-evergreen forests in Ghats (Assam), Karnataka State, in southern India.

12.3 The species of *Hopea* Roxb. are morphologically may be divided into two sections-Euhopes, the secondary nerves not more than 20 pairs, not approximate; and Dryobalanoides, the secondary nerves numerous, approximate, often obscure. Further. the species broadly differ by characteristics of the calyces. H. odorata Roxb. and **W. parviflora** Seddome. have grey tomentose calyx; whereas *Hopea wightiana* Wall has glabrous calyx. There are other several species found in Inida and adjacent regions carry both characters of calyces of lowers in *Hopea* species.

Relevantly *Hopea parviflora* Beddome falling in the group of species with grey-tomentose calyx, differs from *H. cdorata* Roxb. by petals not ciliate, anthers small orbicular, ovary and stylopodium glbrous, stigma 3-fid, stylopodium avoid, and constricted at base.

12.4 Another species of *Hopea* may also be indicated : *Hopea beiferi* (Dyer) Brandis. *Vatica beiferi* Dyer. *Shorea beiberi* (Dyer) Kurz.

12.5 Hopea Roxbnrgḥ nom. cons. species are generally with stipules deciduous and-small; inflorescence a panicle of racemes, axillary or terminal; calyx with 2 lobes enlarging; stamens 10-15; filaments obscurely connate at base; anthers globose; connective produced into a conspicuous own; stigmas thick; and fruits nut-like, enclosed in calyx tube, with 2 lobes accrescent.

Hopea wightiana wall ex wight is distinguishable easily by the echinate axillary and extra-axillary gall-like excrescences.

12.6 The plants of *Hopea* Roxb. are medicinally useful and economically useful also, particularly *Hopea odorata* Roxb. and *H. wightiana* Wall. are utilsed for various purposes.

Hopea odorata Roxb, yields resin (as in *Hopea* trees the resin ducts in the pith 8-12 at the base of a half-bearing internode, and the 2. lateral leaf traces run a short distance only through the bark). Resin of the plant is used as styptic medicine in powder form. Bark is artringent and useful in ailments. Plant produces copal-like resin.

The woods of *Hepea wightiana* Wall ex Wight are strong and used commercially.

13. KLINNAJVĪVĀ-CATUṢKOṆIKĀ-BAHUKUSUMĀ-NIRDAMŚINĪ-ARŚAHARĪ

H13. *Hoppea dichotoma* Hayne ex Willd.

Gentianaceae

Lora, Ramjeeta

Erect, widely branched from the base, annual herbs, 5-15 cm. tall. Stems tetrasgonous. Leaves sessile, ovate-elliptic er-lanceolate, acute, glabrous, 1-narved, 0.3-0.5 x 0.1-0.5 cm., uppermost smaller, passing into bracts. Flowers numerous, in leafy, paniculate cymes. Pedicels 0.05 cm. long. Calyx ribbed, 0.3 cm long, lobes 4, lanceolate, acute. Corolla greenish yellow; lobes 4, ovate-triangular, acute, 0.06-0.8 cm. long. capsule c.2 cm. long.

September to November, October to December.

Throughout India.

13.1 Hoppea dichotoma Willd.

Tiny herbs. Leaves 0.6 X 0.4 cm., evate. Corolla larger than calyx, white.

India. Common in open moist places in plains and upper Ghats, Karnataka State in southern India.

13.2 Hoppea dichotoma Willd. Syn. *Pladera pusilla* Roxb. A small erect glabrous, annual, 2-5 in. high, capiously brancing from near. the base. Stems and branches 4-angled and more or less winged. Leaves about 1/4 in. long, evate, acute. Bracts lanceolate. Calyx 1/10-1/4 in. long, lobes scarious, longer then the corolla, ovate, acuminate, with a prominent green nerves along the margins. Corolla white or pale yellow, ventricose in fruit; lobes half as long as the tube, trinagular, recurved. Capsules ellipsoid. common in Punjab Plains, and in Bengal, Bombay, Central and Southern India. Also in lower Burma, extending to the Philippines.

13.3 Hoppea dichotoma Willd. Plant abundant especially in damp ground. Common in grassy, sandy localities, fields and roadsides in Siwalik region (Dehradun in Uttar Pradesh). Northern India.

13.4 Hoppea fastigiata (Griseb.) G. B. Clarke.

Gentianacae

Tiny herbs. stem 4-winged. Leaves 0.5 x 0.3 cm., ovate. Corolla longer than calyx, white.

October or autumn seasen.

Central and Southen Idia, Sri Lanka. Occasienal in open, grasslands on Ghats, Karnataka state.

13.5 Two species of *Hoppea* Willdenow are distinguishable. *Hoppea dichotema* Willd. has 4-angled stem and with corella included; whereas *H. fastigiata* (Griseb.) C. B. Clarke is also with angled but corolla exserted.

Both are Indian species and their annual herbs are confined to Southern India, with one extending throughout India, ascending up to 990 metres in the mountainous regions.

13.6 In general *Hoppea* Willd. are small, much branched glabrous hamherbs or mostly tiny herbs, with sessile, small, opposite leaves, and the flowers sessile or shortly pedicelled in 2-3 chotomous cymes inflorescence axillary or terminal. Flowers 4-merous, irregular; with clayx campanulate, loves 4, ovate, acuminate, and calyx semotimes lenger than the corolla; corolla with unequal lobes, urcelate tubular, shorter thanm the calyx; stamens perfect and 3 sterile, attached to the threat of the corolla filaments short and linear; anthers small, ovate, dehisching intersely by longitudinal slits, those of the barren stamnes small or nene, rarely with 3 staminodes; every globose or ellipsoid, bivalved, many-seeded, nearly black, obsourely reticulate.

13.7 Whole plant of *Hoppea dischotema* Willd. is madicinally useful, and used in different ailments.

Herb is used in piles and anake bite. Whole plant is pounded and applied over venomous stings. External application is suggested in pile cases.

Plant is considered a antidote to snake bites, and used accordingly in snake bitten cases.

Hoppea and *Hopea* are quite different genera belonging to the families Gentianaceae and Dipterocarpaceae respectively; and former is herb when latter is tree in habit. Species of *Hopea* Roxburgh are separately given in presont context.

14. RATNAPURUṢA-MADANAMATTĀ-RAKTAKUSUMA-GRANTHĀṆUPARṆĪ-LOHITAPUṢPAKĀ

H14. Hybanthus enneaspermus (Linn.) F. Muell.

Ionidium enneaspermus (Linn.) Vent.

I. suffruticosum Ging.

I. heterophyllum Vant.

I. hexapermum Dalz.

Viola suffruticosa.

V. enneaspermus.

Violaceae

Ratan-purus (Hindi), Nunbera (Bengla), Orilatt tamarai (Tamil), Nilakebari (Telugu); Madan-Mastak, Orielaithamarai.

Glabrous or pubescent. Branches diffuse, wooly. Leaves 1.5-2 in., sub-sessile, linear-or lanceolate, serrate; stipules subulate, gland-tipped. Flowers solitary, red; pedicels shorter than the leaves. Petals variable, four of them oblong, acute or mucronate, the fifth with a long claw and a large oval or orbicular limb. Seeds striate.

Different months, June to December.

Bengal and southward to Ceylen. Tropical Asia, Africa and Australia.

14.1 Hybanthus enneaspermus (Linn.) F. Muell.

Annual-perennial herbs, with a woody base. leaves subsessile, linear-lanceolate. stipules subulate, glandtipped. Flowers red, solitary. petals unequal. Seeds striated.

Uttar Pradesh (Bundelkhand, Agra and other parts), Delhi, Bengal, almost throughout the Madras state, Gujarat, Khandesh and Carnatic region.

14.2 Hybanthus enneaspermus (l.) F. V. Muell. Fruticose branching herbs. Leaves up to 3. x 0.2 cm., linear-lanceolate, shallowly crenate. pedicel jointed near bracteoles above middle. Flowers pink. The lowermost petal largest with an elongate, spurred claw toward base and an obovate, broad limb above. seeds striate.

Africa to Australia. Common in dry rock-sand terrain in plains, Karnataka state.

14.3 Various parts of plant *Hybanthus enneaspermus* F. Muell. are medicinally useful.

Plant is toxic and diuretic. Leaves and tender stalks are demulcent.

Roots are used in bowel complaints of children. Fruits are considered conunter against scorpion-sting. Plant contains alkaloids.

The roots of plant *Hybanthus enneaspermus* F. Muell. syn. *Ienidium enneaspermum* DC. are used in asthma. Roots are also useful in pleurisy.

Plant is useful in dysentery and syphilis. It is also useful in impotency.

Leaves are useful in liver complaints Roots are useful in gonorrheea.

15. TIKTAVIṬAPA-SITAPUṢPĀ-PAKṢABĪJĀ-DVIKOKṢṬHAPHALĀ-JVARABANDHIKĀ

H15. *Hymenodictyon orixense* (Roxb.) Mabb.

Hymenodictyon excelsum (Rexb.) Wall.

Cinchono excelsa Roxb.

C. thyrsiflera Roxb.

Rubiaceae

Lamkana (Merwara), Kukurkait, Bhaulan; Barthum (Kangra); Bhaulan, Bhurkul, Kukurkat (Hindi), Dondre (Cujrati), Bhersal (Marathi), Pottaka (Telugu), Kusan(Burmese), Kala hadu (Bombay), Barthen (Punjabi), Sagappu (Tamil), Bandaru (Telugu); Bommal, Bherkud, Mach;

Kodem, phurkhundi, Bhurkhundi(Assam), Inglengalleidho-arong, to-kehe-arong (Mik.), Bon-homjeng (Kachar), Chai-beng-thing, (Kuki, Kal-badom (Mech.), Ding-delebong-sir (Khasi), Bedi-kiruchangipa, Uakundi, Boldikam, Mebol (Gare), Baja-phuty (Kamrup), Lati-karum (Nepali), Uthsmban (Manipur), Boinga (Uattar Pradesh-Kumaon).

Large deciduous tree. Leaves turning yellowish before falling. Bark brownish-grey, smooth on branches and poles, soft and

Large deciduous tree. Leaves turning yellowish before falling. Bark brownish-grey, smooth on branches and poles, soft and corky on old stems; inside softly fibrous; light-dun with bread distant white streaks, 1 in. thick. leaves 4-9 by 2.5-5 in., elliptic-ovate or obovate-oblong, acuminate, membranous, pubescent; lateral nerves 7-10 on either half; base narrowed into the petiole or soute; petiole 1-3 in. long; stipules oblong, with a bread base, caduceus, usually glandular-serrate. Flowers white, fragrant, 2-3 in long, densoly crowded on terminal branched panciles; bracteooles minute; pedicels slander, Calyx minute, pubescent; segments deciduous, acute. corolla pubscent, outside; tube mover than 3 times the length of calyx lobes, slender; limb cup-shaped; lobes 5, valvate, stamens 5, inserted below the throat of the corolla; filaments dilated upwards. Ovary 2-colled, ovules many, style slender, long-exerted; stigma capitate. Capsules elipsoid, 6-1 in. long, reddish-brown when ripe, on recurved pedicels, 2-valved, many seeded. seeds many, lenticular, winged all round; wing deeply cleft at the base.

June to August and October to December.

Base of the Himalayas or sub-Himalayan tracts and Western Himinsula Frequent in the Sal forests in Sub-Himalayan tract, also in Savannahs, from the Ravi eastwards, Bihar, Central Provinces. Deciduous forests of the Peninsula and Burma, Central Previnces Upper and Lower; Cochinchina, Tonkin, Java.

15.1 **Hymenodictyon excelsum** Wall.

Large deciduous tree. Leaves elliptic, blade 4-10, narrowed into petiole 2-4 in. long. Flower pedicellate, white, fragrant in danse cvlindrical compound racemes in terminal drooping panicles. With linear or lanceolate bracts as long as or longer than flower, corolla tube slender, more than three times the length of calyx-lobes. Capsules us to 1 in., on recurved pedicels 1/4 – 1/2 in. long.

Assam province; Kamrup, Newgeng, N. C. Kills, Sibsagar and Cachar.

15.2 **Hymenodictyon obovatum** Wall.

Rubiaceae

green, conspicuous. Flowers sessile, Corolla white. Capsule erect, brown, 2 cm. long.

November to February.

South Western India Rare in Lower Shiradi Ghat, Karnataka; Southern region.

15.3 Hymenodictyon excelsum Wall. Large deciduous tree. Bark of trunk furrowed and rough, that of branches smooth. Leaves 4-10 in. Long by 3-6 in. wide, ovate-elliptic or suborbicular obtuse or abruptly acuminate, narrowed into a petiole 1-3 in., membranous, finely pubscent on both surfaces; lateral nerves, 7-10 pair; atipules oblong, broad-lobed, recurved, usually glandular-serrate, caducous. Floral leaves 3-5 in. long, on long petioles, strongly norved. Flowers many, on the spicate branches of large often drooping pubescent bracteate panicles, small, white or greenish, fragrant; petiole short, bracts large, persistent. Calyx pubescent. Corolla hairy outside, broadly companulate, with short acute lobes. Styles exerted. Capsules on thick decurved pedicels, ellipsoid. Seeds small, many.

Along the base of the Punjab Himalayas east to the Ravi ascending to 5,000 ft.. Siwalik range and foot hills (Dehradun) mainly in salf forests, in Subhimalayan tracts, eastern Uttar Pradesh and also in Merwar (Rajsthan).

15.4 **Hymenodictyon flaccidum** Wall.

Rubiaceae

Pinchwa (Uattar Pradesh-Garhwal)

A dociduous shrub or small tree up to 3 ft. girth and 20 ft. high. pinkish-brown, rough, exfoliating in irregular woody scales. Blaze .3-.5 in., not fibrous, pale yellow mottled and streaked with orange and darkening on exposure. Leaves opposite, 6-10 by 3.5-6 in., broadly elliptic, abruptly short-acuminate, base acute, glabreus above, glabrous or finely pubescent beneath, when young, glossy dark green above, paler and somewhat glossy beneath; with 8-10 pairs of secondary nerves. Petiole 1-2.5 in. long, anther deeply channelled above, Flowers .15 in. long, greenish-yellow, crowded in drooping, spiciform, axillary, simple (rarely branched) pedunculate racemes, 3-8 in. long, usually bearing a single foliaceous persistent bract at the top of the peduncle. Bracts much smaller than the leaves, long petioled. Stamens short. Styles nearly twice the length of the corolla. Capsules .4-.5 in. Long, narrowly ellipsoid, reddish-brown with pale spots, on about pedicels ultimately reflexed surrounded by an elongate membarneous wing. Plant occurring throughout the Uttar Pradesh hills in Kumaon region between 2,000 ft. and 4,500 ft. in scarce frequency. Elsewhere it is also frequently epiphytic on trees. It is frequently growing in cervice amongst rocks in hilly and plant flowers in summers or May to June and fruits in spring season.

15.5 **Hymenodictyon excelsum** Wall.

A medium-sized or large deciduous tree up to 10 ft. girth and 60 ft. height. Bark dark grey or blackish in parts and pale or silvery-grey in parts, rough divided fup into small polygonal rather corky scales. Blaze .5-1.5 in.; pale yellow mottled with orange or brown, the whole somewhat darkening en exposure. Leaves opposite, 4-10 by 3-5 in., elliptic. ovate or obovate-oblong, abruptly acuminate, membranous, pubesent on both surfaces, base narrowed, with 7-10 pairs of secondary nerves; leaves on petiole 1-3 in. long. Flowers .2-.3 long, greenish, fragrant, crowded on the spiciforrm branches of erect terminal panicles 6-10 in. long, the lower one or more pairs of branches usually subtended by foliaceous persistent bracts which resemble the leaves but smaller and long.petiolod. Capsules .5-.7 in. long, ellipsoid, on stout pedicels ultimately reflexed; with seeds surrounded by a membranous reticulate wing.

Plant occurring throughout the Uttar Pradesh hills, Kumaon region, between the areas at 1,000 to 4,000 ft.; and common in dry misceltaneous forests in the hills, often only a small tree. It is flowering in the period of summer to rains and frruiting in winter to Spring.

15.6 The foregoing two species of *Hymenedictyon* Wall. Having trees or shrubs with bitter bark, stipules interpetiolar, deciduous; flowers small 1-2 large leafy reticulate perlsiste bracts and fruits a lecullicidaly 2-valved capsule with winged seeds in general), may be distinguishable in particular. Racemes panicled, erect and leaves puhescent shove in *Hymenodictyon excelsum* Wall.; whereas the leaves glabrous above and recemes simple (rarely branched) drooping in *H. flaccidum* wall.

15.7 The plants *Hymenodictyon excelsum* Wall. is medicinally useful and various parts are used as medicines. They are also of economic uses and employed in veterinary or animal husbandry purposes.

The inner bark of the plant is febrifuge and astringent. Plant contains toxic alkaloid hymenodictine, bitter substance aesculin.

The roots of *Hymenedictyon orixense* (Rexb.) Mobb. syn. *H. excelsum* (Raxb.) Wall. are abortifacient. They are useful in gout, inflammation, and oedema.

Plant is costidered useful in atrophy and carbuncle. It is useful to lactation. Plant is considered useful in pox and sores. Plant useful in cholera.

Bark and reets are febrifuge and used in fever. Bark is specially used in malarial fever.

Bark in the form of decocction or powder is given in liver complaints and febrile conditions.

Bark is useful in females for their menstrual disorders. Roots are given against snake bite. Bark is also useful in diarrhoea.

Leaves are edible and used as vegetable.

The leaves afford fodder for cattles.

The woods are very light and soft, and utilised forr making light and small items. Bark is useful in tannin. leaves are also considered good fodder for buffaloes and other cattles.

16. KHARAKĀṆḌIKĀ-DHAVALASUMANĀ-VṚNTAPATRĀ-VIKṢAT

L16. Lagascea mollis Cav.

Noccaea mollis Jacq.

Asteraceae (cempostae)

Phukri, Kerivapatta

Rigid annual. Stem and branches scabrid. Leaves opposite or the upper alternate, petioled, ovate, acuminate, subcrenate, milky tomentose beneath. Heads in leafy balls, solitary terminating in slender naked; peduncles. Flowers white. Involucral-tubular of 5 connate bracts, anther bases sagitate, auricles obtuse. Style arms elongate, acute, hairy. Achenes cuneate, compressed or 3-angled, tip rounded, pappus very obscure.

Round the year of different seasons; May to September. Running wild in various parts of country. Introduced in India and various warm countries. Indigenous in Central America.

16.1 *Lagascea mollis cav.* Much branched, slender annual herb with scabrid branches. Leaves petioled, ovate. acuminate, sub-crenate silkly tomentose beneath. Clusters of heads solitary terminating in slender naked peduncles. Flowers white; pappus very obscure. Heads in chusters (resembling. simple heads) - 1 in diam., involucrate by elliptic leaves very silky. Upper Gangetic Plains, a weed in cultivated places.

16.2 *Legascia mollis Cavanilles.* A procumbent herb with stem grooved and glbbrous below. Petiole up to 2.5 cm.; leaf-blade 1.5-5 x 1-2.5 cm., ovate, acute, grey-pubescent. Florets white.

Introduced and occurring in various warmer regions of India. common weed in open country in plains, Karnataka, southern India.

16.3 The leaves of plant *Lagascea mollis* Cav. are pounded and applied over wounds, cuts and ulcers leaves are also considered useful in ear complaints.

17. KṢUPAGANDHĀ-DANTURAKĀṆḌĀ-KHARAPATRĀ-NĪLĀRUṆAPUṢPĀ-SAUMANASYĀ

L17. Laggera pterodonta (DC.) Bentham ex C.B. Clarke.

Laggera crispata (Vahl.) Hep. & WD.

Laggera pterodonta Benth.

Blumea pterodonta DC.

Serratula polygona A. Rich.

Blumea pterodonta DC.

Conyza cornua Wall.

Asteraceae

Nhana

Erect, much-branched, strongly aromatic, viscid, annual or perennial herbs, 50-200 cm. tall. stems narrowly winged by the decurrent leaf-bases, gland-hairy or densely pubescent; wings dentate to pinnatifid or pinnatipartite. Leaves obovate or oblong, subacute, apiculate, crispy-hairy, glandular, serrate-dentate;

lower ones long-petioled, often lyrate-pinnatified; upper ones sessile, smaller, 2-15 x 0.3-5 cm. Heads numerous, on 1.5-5 cm. long, pubescent peduncles, in terminal, leafy. corymbiform panicles, 0.5-0.7 cm. across. Peduncles often nodding. Involucre campanulate; bracts 3 to 4-seriate, linear, acute, gland-harry often the inner ones with purplish tips, 0.3-1 cm. long. Marginal flowers 0.7-0. 0.8cm, long, with purplish corollas. Disk-flowers 0.5-0.7 cm. long, with purplish corollas, corolla-lobes gland-hairy. Achenes long-haiy, 0.08-0.1 cm. long. pappus-hairs white, 0.5 cm. long. February to May; January to March. India, Tropical Himalayas, from Shimla, 4,000 ft. elevation eastwards; Assam.

17.1 Leggera pterodonta (DC.)Sch. - Bip. ex Oliv.

Herb, much-branched, glabrous or puberulous, stem with deeply toothed lobed or interrupted wings, leaves sessile oblanceolate toothed or pinnatifid at base, heads 2/3 in. diam, on (usually) slender peduncles at the ends of branches; flowers purple.

Siwalik range, sub-Himalayan tract, Uttar Pradesh. Not uncommon, in damp, shady localities of revines and river banks and other areas.

17.2 Leggera pterodonta (DC.) Eentham ex C.B. Clarke. Viscid herbs to 1.5 m.; wing on stem toothed. Leaves up to 10 x 4 cm., elliptic, acute at tip, decurrent on to stem wing, crenate. Heads few-solitary. Florets purple. Achenes ribbed. Tropical Africa, Burma, India. Fairly common in upper Ghats, along roadsides, and, outskirts of wet deciduous forests, Karnataka

17.3 Laggera alata (D. Den) Sch.-Bip ex oliv

Erigeron alatum D. Don.

Vernonia wightiana Wall.

Conyza alata Roxb.

Blumea alata DC.

Conyza nutans Blume.

Laggera divaricata Oliv.

Blumea vernonioides DC.

Asteraceae (Composiate)

Robust much-branched leafy perennial herb, pubescent or tomentose and sometimes glandular. Stems 2-4 ft., with broad entire wings. Leaves sessile, 1-4 in., long, narrowly oblong, acute, denticulate or subentire, rough above, woolly beneath, decurrent on the stem at thier base. Heads small, racemed on the wings axillary branches, nodding in fruit. Involucral-bracts many; outer short, herbaceous, often recurved, inner longer an straight. Flowers purplish corolla of outer slender. Achenes apporessedly hairy Pappus white.

September to October; November-December.

Tropical Himalayas up to 5,000 ft. elevation from Simla to Sikkim and in the hilly region of Central and Southern India to Ceylon and Burma.

17.4 Laggera alata (B.Ion.) Sch.-Sip ex Oliver syn.*Blumea alata* D. Don.) DC.

Erect, pernnial herbs, stems glandular-pubescent. Leaves sessile, oblong, acute, denticulate or subentire, woolly beneath. Heads arranged in leafy racemes. Outer involucral bracts herbaceous, often recurved; inner ones longer and erect. corallas purplish. Achenes appressed-hairy. Pappus hairs white.

Siwalik range; Hill regions throughout India, within 300-2000 m. elevation. Himachal Pradesh, Sutlej and Giri vallyes.

17.5 Blumea alata (D. Don.) DC.

Laggeralata (D.Den.) C. Schultz ex Oliver. An erect, pubescent annual herbs upto 90 cm, high. stem lesfy, robust, Broadly winged with decurrent leaf-bases. Leaves alternate, sessile, oblong, acute, teeth numerous, small and sharp,oblong-lanceolate, decurrent on to wing of stem, dentate, glandular. Heads discoid, many in axillary racemes, often forming large, terminal leafy panicles or racemose panicles; peduncles and outer bracts of involucre bracts many, acute, outer shorter, inner equalling the flowers. Pappus white. Flowers purple, corollas of the outer very slender, of inner larger, 5-lobed. Achenes small, hairy. Paleotropics. India, Java, China, Philippines Islands, Tropical Africa, Madagascar, Ceylon, Burma. Southern India, Karnataka.

17.6 Laggera flava (DC.) Bentham ex C.B. Clarke.

Blumea flava DC.

Blumeopsis flava (DC) Gagnep.

Erigeron falcatum Don.

Asteraceae (Composite)

Slender glabrous or puberulous herb 6 in. to 3 ft. high. stem simple or corymbosely branched above, sulcate. Leaves 1-3 in. long, lower petioled; cauline, semi-ampleticaul, ovate-lanceolate or obovate, sharply dentate or incised or sometimes almost entire, membranous, glaucous or subscabrous. Heads few, small, on the slender branches of loose panicled cymes. Outer invol-bracts ovate, acute; inner longer, lanceolate, acuminate, all glabrous or with ciliate margins. Receptacle glabrous. Flowers golden-yellow; lobes of horn, corolla glabrous; anthers. sagitate. Achenes very minute, glabrous. Pappus white.

Cold season.

Outer Himalayas up to 6,000 ft. elevation from Uttar Pradesh hills to Sikkim and Bhutan and in the hilly parts of Bengal, Central and Southern India. Burma and Malay Peninsula.

17.7 Laggera flava (DC.) Bentham ex C ? B. Clarke. A herb upto 40 cm. stem terete, grooved, glabrous. Leaves up to 8 x 4 cm. obovate-oblong, cordate-sagitate and amplexicaul at base, serrate-dentate. Heads in panicles. Flowers yellow. Achenes ribbed.

India, eastwards to Burma. and Sikkim and Bhutan). Occasional in dry deciduous forests, Karnataka.

17.8 **Laggera aurita** suh. - Bip. ex C.B. clarke

Conyza aurita Linn. f.

Blumea aurita DC.

Asteraceae

Soanputru (Mundari)

Perennial herb, viscidly pubescent or villous. Stem up to 3 ft. high, erect, cylindrical, not winged. leaves sessile or petioled, 2-4 in. long on the main stem, the upper smaller and bract-like, oblanceolate, subacute, toothed lobed or semi-pennatifid, shortly decurrent. Heads small, arranged in terminal panicled corymbs. Involucral bracts slender, linear, acute, spftly villose; inner longer, scarious. Receptacle glabrous. Flowers pink. Achenes hairy, dark red.

February to March

Punjab Plains and Bengal south to Travancore, eastward to Chittagong and Burma, extending to tropical Africa.

17.9 Laggera aurita Schultz. A slender (or rather slender), viscidly hirsute or villous herb, 0.3-0.9. m. high, pubescent or villous, stem not winged; leaves small sessile or petioled oblanceolate toothed lobed cut or half-pinnatifid; heads 1/4 – 1/2 in. in diam. in small lateral, terminal corymbose; flowers pink or purplish.

Waste place from Punjab eastwards to West Bengal, Orissa, Andhra Pradesh, Madras, Kerala and Bombay. Upper Gangetic Plains, abundant within the area.

17.10 The plants of *Laggera* sch. -Bip. are medicinally useful and chemically potent.

The plant of *Laggera aurita* Sch-Bip. is strongly scented and produces the odour of turpentine. The leaves are considered useful to stop bleeding from cuts as the plant has styptic action.

Laggera alata Sch.-Bip is considered useful as a disinfectant. Tender leaves appearing after the rains (first) have the odour of black currant and reported to yield on ethereal oil. Whole plant of *Laggera crispat* Vahl.) Hep. & Wd. syn. Lagger *L. pterodonta* Benth. is considred useful in blood pressure.

18. GOJIKĀ-PĪTASRAVĀ-DANTURADALĀ-BAHUPUṢPAŚĀKHĪ-DUGDHADĀTRĪ

L18. Launaea nudicaulis Hook. f.

Lactuaca obtusa Clarke.

Prenanthes procumbens Roxb.

Alcorhynchus nudicaulis Less.

Asteraceae (Composiate).

Balthal, Dudhlak (Punjabi), Akria, Ban gobhim, Jangli Gobhi (Rajsthan), Pathari (Bombay)

Glabrous, biennial or perennial herb, with yellow juice. Flowering stems ususlly many, about 6 in. long, spreading on all sides. simple or branched, naked or with a few small leaves below the clusters of flowers. Leaves usually sessile, 2-10 in. long, sinuate-lobed, runcinate or pinnatifid; lobes irregularly lobulate and sharply toothed, the teeth usually white and cartilaginous. Heads 1/2 to 1/4 in. long sessile, narrow, in terminal and sub-racemose clusters, rarely solitary. Pedicels scaly with small bracts. Invol-bracts overtopping the pappus with white membranous margin; outer shortly ovate, inner long, linner, with the midrib thickened in fruit. Achenes small or 1/12 in., columnar, thickly ribbed, outer ones compressed, much shorter than the soft whtie pappus.

Cold season.

Plains of Bengal and Punjab, and southwards through Sindh to the Deccan; Western Himalayas upto 6, 000ft. in Kumaon; also in Waziristan and Afghanistan and westwards to the Atlantia.

18.1 Launaea asplenifolia (Billd.) Hook. f.

Prenanthes asplenifolia Willd.

Microrhynchus asplenifolius (Willd.) DC

L. aspleniifolia (Willd.) Hook. f.

Asteraceae

Erect, annual or biennial herbs, usually multicauline, with milky juice. Stems simple or branched at the top, leafless, often ascending or trailing, up to 5-20(30) cm. tall. Leaves in a basal rosette, obovate-oblanceolate, with a narrowed base, pinnatifid or pinnately lobed, 5-10 (-12) cm. long; segments ovate-oblong, remotely denticulate with non-cartilaginous teeth. glabrous. Heads 1-1.5 cm. long, on 0.3-0.8 (1) cm. long, bracteate peduncles, in a terminal panicle. Involucral bracts 2-seriate; outer ones ovate, acute, 0.25-0.3 cm. long, on 0.3-0.8 (-1) cm. long, bracteate peduncles, in a terminal panicle. Involucral bracts 2-seriate, acute, 0.25-0.3 cm. long; inner ones lanceolate acute, 0.8 cm. long. Ligules yellow, of marginal flowers purple-tinged on the back. Achenes not seen. Pappus hairs white, 0.7-0.8 cm.

March to June; Spring to summer season or cold months.

Plains of Punjab and Bengal, an southwards to the Circars; also in the Andaman Islands and in Burma.

18.2 **Launaea nudicaulis** Hook. f. a biennial or perennial herb with a tuft of simple or branched flowering stems arising from a rosette of sessile, lobed or runcinate, sharply toothed leaves (5-25 cm. X 2.5-7.5 cm.) and bearing yellowish flower heads either solitary or in clusters. It occurs as a weed more or less throughout the plains of India, ascending up to an altitude of 2,400 m. in the Himalayas; the Upper Gangetic Plains an Siwaliks, northern and Central India.

18.3 **Launaea asplenifolia** Hook. f. A biennial or perennial herb with long slender roots, narrowly obovate, lobed and toothed leaves and yellow paniculate flower heads. It is found throughout the plains of northern India and Bengal extending southwards to Andhra Pradesh; also in Andamans. Upper Gangetic plains, Siwaliks, northern and central India. Sandy, grassy localities and fields and other areas.

18.4 **Launaea acaulis** (Roxb.) Babcock ex Craib.

Crepis acaulis (Roxb). Hook, f.

Prenanthes acaulis Roxb.

Asteraceae

Erect, perennial herbs, often multicauline, with a thick, stout, long, cylindrical taproot. Stems simple or branched in the upper part, glabrous, with milky juice. Leaves in a radical rosette, linear-lanceolate or narrowly oblong, with a narrowed base, acute or remotely denticulate, glabrous, up to 6-12 (-15) X 1-1.5 cm. Heads 10-12 flowered, on 1-1.5 cm. long, bracteate peduncles, in terminal panicles, 1.3-1.8 cm. long. Involucral bracts 3 seriate; outer ones ovate; inner ones labceolate. acute. Ligules 1.8-2 cm. long, yellow, 3-dentate, glabuous. Achenes ellipsoid, ribbed, contracted at the top, narrowed at both ends, 0.6-0.7 cm. long. Pappus-hairs white.

Spring to summer season; February to May

Subtropical Himalayas from Japan to Bhutan, Bengal, Central and South India; and in Shah hills in Burma.

The species is more closely allied to *Crepis* Linn. rather than to *Launaea* Cass., as the habit, inflorescence, involucres and achenes render it more like a species of *Crepis* Linn.

18.5 Crepis acaulis Hook if.

Prenanthes acaulis Roxb.

Glabrous stemless, perennial herb. Root woody, straight, cylindric. Leaves chiefly radical, 2-12 in. long, lanceolate linear or narrowly obovate-spathulate, obtuse or acute, entire sinuate-toothed or, subpinnatifid nerves spreading, faint. Scape 4-or 5 flowered, usually shorter than the leaves, 8-10 in. long, simple or dichotomously branched. Heads, few, 1 in. long, 10-12 -flowered; peduncles bracteolate. Outer involucre bracts very small; inner linear, the margins haline. Flowers yellow, pedicelled. Achenes small or 2/4 in. about, ellipsoid, subcompressed, shorter than the soft silvery pappus, ribs smooth.

Central and Southern India, subtropical Himalayan regions; Upper Gangetic Plains, Siwaliks range, Dehradun, North Oudh, eastern Uttar Pradesh and other adjoining States, Grassy, sandy localities waysides, first edges, forest clearings an other areas.

18 6 Launaea procumbens (Roxb.) Ramayya & Rajagopal.

Prenanthes procumbens Roxb.

Launaea nudicaulis auct. pl. (India), non. Hook, f. sens. strict

Microrhynchus nudicaulis (Linn.) Loss. non

Chondrilla nudicaulis L. non

Asteraceae

Perennial herbs, multicauline, with yellow juice. Root stout, thick, woody. Stems simple or sparingly branched, erect or scandent or trailing or scrambling over other plants. Leaves in a basal rosette, oblong-oblanceolate or spathulate, with a narrowed base, obtuse, repand-denate to pinnately lobed or pinnatified, somewhat glancous beneath, 5-20 cm. long; lobes closely denticulate with cartilaginous teeth. Heads yellow, 1.5 cm. long, on 0.5-1 cm. long, bracteate peduncles, solitary or in clusters, combined into a terminal, subracemose inflorescence. Iinvolucral bracts 3-seriate. outer ones ovate, 0.3-0.2 cm. long; inner ones lanceolate, 0.5-1 cm. long. Ligules yellow; marginal ones purplish on the back. Achenes rugulose, ribbed, 0.35-0.4 cm. long, Pappus-hairs white, with a pappiferous disk, 0.8 cm. long.

Spring to Autumn season; March to November or December. Upper Gangetic Plains, Siwalik range, Dehradun. Grassy, sandy localities, roadsides, gardens, river-beds, fields, forest edges, forest clearings and scrub jungles.

18.7 **Launaea fallax** (Jaub and Spanch) O. K.

Launaea nudicaulis Hook. f.

Microrhychus nudicaulis (Linn.) Loss **M. fallax** Jaub.

Astenaceae

Perennial herb, multicauline, with yellow juice. Root stout, thick and woody. Stems simple or sparingly branched, erect or trailing or scrambling over other plants. Leaves in a basal rosette, oblong-oblanceolate or spathulate, with a narrowed base, obtuse, repand, dentate to pinnately lobed or pinnatifid, somewhat glaucous beneath, 5-20 cm. long, lobes closely denticulate with cartilage-pointed teeth. Heads yellow, 1.5 cm. long, on 0.5-1 cm. long bracteate peduncles, solitary or in clusters, combined into a terminal subracemose inflorescence; involucral bracts 3-seriate; ligules yellow, marginal ones with purplish bracts; achenes rugolose, pitted, 0.35-0.4 cm. long; pappus hairs with a pappifeous disk, 0.8 cm. long.

March to November

Upper Gangetic plains and Siwalik range, Dehradun.

Earlier the species was associated with *Microrhynchus nudicaulis* (Linn.) Less., but it is later considered to be distinct from it.

18.8 **Launaea residifolia** (Linn.) Druce.

Scorzonera residifolia Linn.

Zollikoferia chondriotilloides DC.

Asteraceae

Perennial glabrous herb with little milky sap, 3-8 cm. high. Stem dichotomously branched, terete, sulcate, woody at base. Radical leaves sub-rosulate, 4-15 X 5-2 cm., lanceolate or runcinate-pinnatifid, spinolose-toothed, attenuate at base, cauline sessile, half-amplexicaule, narrower and pinnatifid, ovate or deltoid at froks of peduncles, entire, apparently bracts-like. Heads 1-2 cm. long on subdivaricate, bracteate peduncles. Involucral bracts 3-4 seriate with 3-4 bracts in each series; ligules of marginal flowers on outer surface greyish an with two parallel purple veins. Pappus white, longer than achenes, inner few visibly longer and rigid than the numerous soft outer hairs. Achenes 6-7 mm. long, narrowly cylindric, slightly contracted below the apical truncate end at base obscurely 3-4 toothed, strongly ribbed, the ribs scarbulous, receptacle naked.

Throughout the year, specially in summer season.

Punjab, Multan, hills of Rawalpindi, Sindh, Persia, Afghanistan, Arabia and Egypt. Rajasthan in India.

18.9 **Launaea acaulis** (Roxb.) Babe. Perennial herb with subterranean, short stem. Leaves rosulate, 2-6 X 1-2 cm., obovate, lanceolate, acute or rounded at tip, narrowed but amplexicaule at base, glaucous beneath, entire, distantly toothed to runcinate. Heads few-many, bracts 1-3-seriate, herbaceous, oblong-lanceolate. Corolla bright yellow, 1-8 cm. long. Achenes cylindrical, truncate at both ends ribbed, glabrous.

January to May.

India is China. Plains and Upper Ghats, Karnataka, Southern India.

18.10 **Launaea glomerata** Hook. f. Glaucescent herb with lobed, pinnatifid or runciate leaves, yellow flower heads and conspicuously winged fruit. It is found in Kathiawar, Kutch and Mount Abu in Gujarat and Rajasthan.

18.11 **Launaea sarmentosa** (Bl.) Kan.

Prenanthes sarmentosa Cass.

Lactuca sarmentosa DC.

L. sarmentosa (Willd.) Alston.

Microrhynchus sarmentosa DC.

Asteraceae

Pathri (Bombay), Bhonpatri (Marathi), Bombay (Hindi), Bhonapatri (Gujarati) Glabrous herb. Leaves runcinate-pinnatifid or sinuate-toothed or lobed, 1-3 in., rarely more, teeth rarely white and cartilaginous. Flowering stems slender, 1-3 ft. long, arching from node to node, procumbent, long flageliform rooting and leafing at the nodes, heads of the nodes solitary or clustered, short, usually with bracteate peduncles. Involucral bracts almost 3-seriate, with white membranous margins, outer short, intermediate longer, inn or linear midrib at the base hardening in fruit. Achenes columnar very thickly ribbed much shorter than the soft straight white pappus, small, pale, usually obtusely 4-gonous; pappus 1/4 in., deciduous, hairs very slender, white and of nearly equal length.

Sandy coasts of India; from Bengal to Ceylon, Penang, Madras and Malabar. Mauritius, Egypt, East African coast. Sandy seas beaches localities in India and also considered as a sand binder plant in certain regions.

18.12 **Launaea glomerata** Cassini.

Lomatolepis glomerata Cass.

Sonchus capitatus Sor.

Microrhynchus glomerata Jaub.

Zollikoferia glomerata Boiss.

Asteraceae

Alko (Quetta)

Glabrous herb. Leaves sessile, sinuate-lobed, pinnatifid or runcinate, lobes usually short rounded toothed, teeth cartilaginous white, lobes or pinules numerous, close set. leaf 3-5 by about one and half inches. Flowering branches stout, strict, usually not exceeding the leaves, naked, spreading sparingly dichotomously branched. Heads broader than in other species (India), with broader 3-seriate more obtuse invol. bracts, and more numerous flowers. Involucral bracts with very broad membranous margins outer large broadly ovate, inner oblong, case hardened in fruit; peduncles short, bracteolate. Achenes corky thickly ribbed outer 2-winged inner columar shorter than the soft straight white pappus, achenes small, pale yellow, outer slightly curved, linear-oblong, emarginate at both ends, wings reach as broad or broader than the nucleus ventrally and dorsally 5-6 ribbed, wings and ribs minutely crenulate; inner achenes often narrower and imperfect.

Punjab, Sindh. Persia, Arabia, Egypt, Algiers.

18.13 Various species of *Launaea* Cass. are distinguishable by their major characteristics, For the instance, the achenes with a contracted top and leaves entire or remotely denticulate are in *Launaea acaulis* (Roxb.) Babe; whereas top and leaves lyrate-pinnatifid are in other two species. which may be separated. Plants are annuals or biennials with milky latex and leaf-segments remotely denticulate in *Launaea asplenifolia* (Willd.) Hook. f., whereas the plants are perennials with yellow latex and leaf-segments closely denticulate in (*Launaea procumbens* (Roxb.) R. & R.

18.14 The characters of flowers also differ in two species. Heads terminal on the paniculately branched flowering stems are in *Launaea asplenifolia* Hook. f.; when heads more or less racemose on the flowering stems and the branches in *Launaea nudicaulis* Hook. f.

The character of achenes in *Launaea* species is also a basic differentiating factor as broadly the achenes are not winged in various species (India) but the achenes are winged in *Launaea glomerata* Cass. The species having non-winged achenes are further distinguished in general on the basis of characters of heads and flowering and separated by various specific characteristics and features of plants.

18.15 Various species of *Launaea* Cass. are medicinally useful and also used in veterinary as well as economic purposes. For several uses, different parts of the plants are employed.

The roots of *Launaea asplenifolia* Hook. f. in combination with other drugs are used as galactogogue.

Whole plant of *Launaea chandrilloides* Hoof. f. are used as galactagogue.

The decoction of whole plant at *Launaea glomerata* Hook. f. mixed with wheat meal is applied as a poultice in sore eye complaints including eyeache.

Whole plant of *Launaea acaulis* (Roxb.) Kerr. is used as galactogogue. Roots are useful in urine complaints.

Whole plant of *Launaea mucronata* (Forsk) Muschler is useful for its galactogoguge properties. Decoction of the roots is also given to remove constipation.

Leaves of *Launaea nudicaulis* Hook. f. are applied to the head of suffering children as a cure of fever. The plant is used as a fodder for goats. It is also used in the preparation of a cooling sherbet. Leaves are used in curries. Leaves are edible as vegetable. The garland of roots is worn to ward off evil spirits as per belief.

Whole plant of *launaea sarmentosa* Alston. is useful in gout. Roots are useful in rheumatism. Plant is considered to possess tonic, sudorfic, diuretic and aperient properties. It is also used as a substitute for Taraxacum. Leaves are eaten also during femine. Herb is fed to buffaloes as a galactogogue.

19. DAṀŚANIKĀ-HARITĀBHAPUṢPTĪ-KAṆḌULA- SAUTRA CARMĀ-DHĀNYABĪJĀ

Laportea crenulata Gaudich.

Laportea stimulus Miq.

Urticaceae

Utigun (Hindu), Chorpata (Bengal), Torash, ṣorot-gach (Assam). Ottapilava (Tamil), Anachoriyan (Malyalam), Thlak-pui (Lushai) Moringe (Nepal), Gilmat-jakma (Garo), Ongyalop (Lepcha), Gernayung (North Cachar), Dieng-syn-rem (Khasi), Phaji (Miri), Kherma-phang (Çachaṟ), Laua-chutra (Sylhet), Paji (Abor.), Tarmepi-arong, Bap kangsan (Mik.), Thakpui-kung (Tip.), Khoma, Phoma (Mech.), Ougyatop.

Herbaceous stemmed shrub; young parts clothed with stinging hairs. Leaves 6-14 by 3-5 inches, ovate or elliptic, more or less entire, sometimes crenulate towards the apex, acute or acuminate, clothed with stinging harirs, penninerved; base rounded or cordate; petiole stout, 1-4 in. long. Urticle inflated, white.

August to December

Tropical Himalayas from Sikkim eastwards, Assam, Khasia hills. Western Ghats of Madras State or Tamilnadu at 1,000 to 5,000 ft. and Rempa hills at 2,500 ft.

19.1 **Laportea crenulata** Gaud. Devil Nettle, Fever Nettle. A large stout shrub or small tree, 3-4 m. high, found growing gregariously in evergreen forests in tropical Himalayas from Nepal eastwards Bihar, Chota Nagpur, North Bengal, plains and hills of Assam; Rampa hills in North Circars, Anaimalai hills and western ghats in Kerala at altitudes of 300-1500 m.

Shrub with white bark, smooth, thin; leaves oval to oblong or oblong-lanceolate; flowers minute, greenish, dioecious, in axillary cymes; achenes small, obliquely ovoid, black, shining.

19.2 **Laportea interrupta** Wight.

Laportea interrupta (Linn.) Chew.

Urtica interrupta Linn.

Fleurya interrupta (L.) Gaud.

Urticaeeae

Erect herb, 10-40 cm. tall, stems flexuous, terete, furrowed; entire plant covered sparingly with stinging hairs. Leaves 3.5-9.5 x 2.3-7.5 cm., broadly ovate, alternate, crenate-serrate along margins, sparingly clothed with bulbous-based stinging hairs on both surfaces, acuminate, cordate, shortly cuneate or sub-truncate at base, 3-nerved petiole 1-8 cm long, slender, hairy; stipules 2.4-5 mm. long, 2-fid at apex, segments linear-subulate. acuminate-aristate at apex. Flowers greenish in distant paniculate cymose monoecious clusters; cymose clusters arranged, 15-16 cm. long interrupted axillary racemes; peduncles 1-5.5 cm. long, grooved, hairy. Male flowers pedicels 0.4-1 mm. long, thick, perianth 1-1.2 mm. long, 4-lobed to the base, stamens 4, inflexed in bud, pistillate clavate. Female flowers pedicels about 0.5 mm. long, 4-toothed, upperteeth hooded, lower minute, each more or less deltoid, cililate along margins, with downwardly curved style at apex, more or less truncate at base, straw-brown.

August to January

Khasi hills, West Beggal, Bihar, Western Peninsula, Ceylon, Madras, Pacific Islands, China, Abyssenia.

19.3 **Fleurya interrupta** (Linn.) Preye

Urtica interrupta Linn.

Urticaceae

Erect or decumbent-ascending, often rooting at base, simple or branched, annual herbs, with stinging hairs. Stems sulcate, purple-at oaked, subglabrous or pilose towards the apex. Leaves ovate, with a subcordate base, acuminate, coarsely serrate, with inconspicuous cystolitis, thinly pilose, 2-15 X 1.5-10 cm, Petiole 1-10 (-15) cm. long. Stipules 2-fid, 0.5-0.6 cm. long. Flower-clusters combined into interrupted, 3-30 cm. long pseudo-spikes, combined into a panicle. Male flowers pedicels 0.08-0.1 cm. long; perianth-segments 4-5, ovate, acute, hairy at the top, 0.12 cm. long; stamens 4-5; pistillode minute. Female flowers subsessile; perianth-segments 4, unequal; style subterminal. Achenes obliquely ovoid, compressed, 0.15 X 0.1-0.13 cm. August to November.

Assam province, Khasi hills; Dehradun, Siwaliks, Uttar Pradesh.

19.4 **Fleurya** Gaud. is sometimes considered as congeneric with

Laportea Gaud. This is distinguished from *Laportea* by linear cystoliths and margined, mostly tuberculate achenes. *Laportea* is characterised by punctate cystoliths and non-margined, smooth achenes.

Fleurya Gaud. is also reduced some times as a section of *Laportea* Gaud.

19.5 **Fleurya interrupta** Gaud. A nettle-like erect herb, with stinging hairs. Leaves with linear cystoliths, alternate, 5-6 in., long, ovate, acuminate, coarsely toothed with bulbous based hair above, glabrous beneath except on the nerves; base 3-nerved; subcordate, truncate or cuneate; petioles longer than the blade; stipules 2-fid. Cytmes 6-14 in long tax; branchlets and pedicles recurved. Male and female on the same clusters. Male 4-5 merous. Female perianth cupular, 4-lobed. Ovary oblique. Achenes oblique. Seeds nearly exalbu, inous.

Autumn season; August to November.

Assam province, Khasi hills.

19.6 **Laportea pterostigma** Wedd.

Urticaceae

Paji-asing (Miri), Pase-gilong (Abour.), Tarme (Mik.), Phepha. soroth (Assamese), Son-rem (Khasi).

Large tree of 60-120 ft. height. Bark whitish with vertical lines of lenticles and distant horizontal wrinkles stem buttressed at base; bark .7 in., thick, very soft white inside; woos very soft. Leaves 8-12 by 0.5-8 in., ovate or broadly, elliptic, more or less entire, acute or somewhat acuminate, subcoriaceous, palminerved; base rounded or truncate; petiole 6-8 in. long, stout.

Colder months to spring seawon.

Assam province, N.E.F. tract

19.7 **Iaportea terminalis** Wight

Urticaeeae

Patle sisnu (Nepalese)

Erect herb, 0.6-1.2 m. high, with orbicular to oblong-ovate or lanceolate leaves.

Sub-tropical Himalayas from Kuman eastwards, North Bengal, Naga and Aka hills in Assam, Nilgiri and Palni hills and Kerala, at altitudes of 1,200-2,700 m. Assam provinces; Naga hills.

19.8 Two species of genus *Laportea* Gaud. are initially separated by habit of plants as *Laportea terminalis* Wight. and

Laportea crenulata Gaud. are herbaceous shrub or erect herb. while *Laportea pterostigma* Wedd. is large tree.

Fleurya interrupta (Linn.) Gaud. is chiefly allied to Fleurya *aestuans* (Linn.) Gaud., but this many be distinguished by flower-clusters being combined into interrupted pseudo-spikes. *Fleurya aestuans* (Linn.) Gaud. is characterised by flower-clusters being combined into flat and dense corymbs.

19.9 Some other species of genus *Laportea* Gaud. may be referred in this context:-

Laportea aestuans (L.) Chew.

Utica aestuans L.

Fleurya cordata Gaud.

F. petiolata Decne.

Laportea bulbifera (Sieb. & Zuce) Wedd.

Urtica bulbifera Sieb. & Zucc.

Laportea terminalis W.

L. oleracea Wedd.

Laportea terminalis Wedd. is treated as distinct from *Laportea bulbifera* Wedd. as the Himalayan plants are not so conspicuously bulbiferous as *L. bulbifera* (Sieb & Z.) Wedd.

19.10 **Dendrocnide sinuata** (B.) Chew.

Laportea crenulata. Wedd.

Urtica sinuata (Bl.) Chew

U. crenulata Roxb.

Dendrocnide meyeniana (Walp.) Chew.

Urtica meyeniana Walp.

Laportea pterostigma Wedd.

It is sometimes concluded in the basis of study of whole group on a monographic basis that *Dendrocnide* to quite distinct from *Laportea* which needs restablishment of its status.

19.11 **Laportea crenulata** Gaud. plant is considered poisonous. Seeds are in the same way as coriander. Juice of the roots is used in long-standing fevers.

The whole plant is clothed with small highly irritant hairs of herbs, the sting of which causes dermatitis and acute burning pain in the body. The effect lasts for several days and is aggravated when water is applied to the affected sting. The sting is particularly powerful during the flowering season when it produces violent sneezing, sleep-lessness and fever.

The juice of the root is considered useful in chronic fevers. Boots and leaves are applied to swellings and blind abscess. The seeds are used medicinally like coriander.

Laportea terminalis right. is medicinally useful. Young shoots are eaten after boiling. The stinging hairs on the plants cause dermatitis.

The plant *Laportea crenulata* Gaudlich. is also economically useful. The stem bark yields a strong fibres (cellulose content 53-54 per cent); length of ultimate cell, 8-16 mm.) used by the hill tribes of Assam for cordage and for making coarse cloth. It is considered to rhea (*Boehmeria rivea)* and is not of any commercial importance because of the presence of stinging heirs which render fibres extraction difficult. Flowers are used in some areas in preparing curries.

20. BHULGNIKĀ-KAKṢAKUSUMĀ-ĀRDRABHŪYĀ-CITRAPUṢPĪ-TVACYĀ

20. Lindernia anagallis (N. Burman) Pennel

Ruellia anagallis N. Burman.

Cratiola pedunculata Bentham.

Lindernia cordifolia (Colsm.) Merrill

Vendellia angustifolia Benth

V. cordifolia (Colsm.) G. Don.

Torenia diffusa Roxb.

Scrophulariaceae

Godagvel (Marathi)

Small diffuse glabrous herb. Stems often creeping at the base and rooting from the nodes, sometimes tinged with purple; branches 4-16 in. long, slender. Leaves shortly stalked, 1/2 – 3/4 in. long, ovate, obtuse or subacute, obscurely crenate-serrate, usually unequally subcordiate at the base. Flowers solitary, pedicels about twice as long as the leaves. Calyx-segments almost free to the base, narrowly lanceolae, acuminate. Corolla 3/4 in. long, white, margined with pale-purple and marked with a yellow spot on the lower lip. Capsule linnear lanceolate, acute, twice as long as the calyx. Seeds ellipsoid.

Rainy and cold seasens; July to November.

Throughout India in Ceylon; Western Himalaya upto 4,000 ft. and extending to the Malay Penisula, Borneo, China and Cochin-china.

20.1 **Vandellia pedunculata Benth.** Erect-ascending or decumbent-ascending, annual herbs. Stems decumbent or creeping, and rooting below, often branched form the base, glabrous. Leaves on 0.15-0.5 cm. long petioles, ovate-oblong, with a rounded or cordate base, subacute or subobtuse, crenate-serrate, glabrous, 1-3 x 0.9-2.3 cm. Flowers axillary, solitary. Pedicels 2-3 cm. long during anthesis, afterwards up to 3 cm. long. calyx 0.5-0.6 cm. long; segments lanceolate, acute. Corollea 1-1.5 cm. long, purple; upper lip entire; lower lip 3-lobed, yellow on the throat. Stamens 4, fertile; anthers basally tailed. Capsule beaked with a persistent style, 1-1.3 cm. long.

Mere or less throughout India, in damp places. Abudant within the areas of Upper Gangeic Plains, Siwaliks and Sub-Himalayan tracts, specially in swamps, rice fields and marshy localities.

20.2 **Lindernia anagallis (N. Burman) Pennel.** Decumbent herbs. Leaves shortly petiolate, ovate, obscurely serrate, truncate-cordate, up to 1.5 x 1 cm. Pedicels axillary, up to 3 cm. Corolla pink. Stamens 4; anterior filaments appendiculate. Fruiting calyx divided almost to base, less than half the lenght of the capsule.

Indomalaysia. Occasional in moist places in Ghats, Karnataka State; Southern India.

20.3 **Lindernia procumbens** (Krock.) Philoox.

Vandellia pyxidaria Linn.

Lindernia parviflora Linn.

Vandellia pyxidaria (Linn.) Maxim.

V. erecta Benth.

Anagalloides procumbens Krock.

Gratiola intergrifolia Roxb.

Scrophulariaceae

Vakapushpi (Bombay, Marathi)

Small erect glabrous annual, 4-8 in. hinh, branching from the base, branches not rooting. Leaves sessile, elliptic or oblong, obtuse, entire or obscurely crenate; nerves 3-5 in. long, parallel. Pedicels axillary, solitary, slender, usually twice as long as the leaves. Calyx-segments 1.8-1/6 in. long, free to the base, lanceolate or linear, Anther obtuse, shorter than the ovoid-orbicular capsule.

Rainy and cold seasons.

Himalayas from Kashmir to Assam; common in Bengal, also in South and Central India; extending to Siam, China, Japan, Malaya and Polynesia and westwards to France.

Vandelia pyxidaria Maxim. plant occurring in Upper Gangetic Plains, Siwaliks (Dehradun), Bundelkhand (Uttar Pradesh).

20.4 **Lindernia antipoda** (Linn.) Alat.

Ruellia antipoda Linn.

Bonnaya veronicifolia (Retz.) Spreng.

Lindernia verbenifolia (Colsm.) Penn.

Hybanthes veronicifolia (Rotz.) Urban. (*'veronicaefolia'*) Scrophulariaceae Prostrate or decumbent-descending, annual herbs. Stems obtusely 4-angular, often branched from the base, creeping and rooting below. Leaves subsessile or short-/etieled, lanceólate-oblong or obovate, narrowed towards the base, subacute, subentire-crenate to serrate, glabrous, 1-5 x 3-.06 cm. Flowers axillary or in leafy racemes. Bracts linear-lanceolate, 0.3-0.35 (-0.5) cm. long. Pedicels during anthesis 0.6-1 cm. long, afterwards 0.8-1.5 cm. long. Calyx divided near to the base; segments linear-lanceolate, serrate in the uper part. Corolla bluish purple, 0.65-1 cm. long. Fertile stamens 2; staminodes yellowish clavate. Capsule cylindric, 1.5 cm. long. seeds 0.03-0.04 x 0.02 cm.

June to December.

Indomalaysia. Frequent in marshy rice-fields of Upper Ghats and Western Plains, Karnataka, Siwaliks in Uttar Pradesh.

20.5 **Lindernia hyssopoides** (1.) Naines.

Lindernia hyssopides (L.) Haines. (*'hyssopioides'*)

Gratiola hyssopides M. (*'hyssopioides'*)

Hybanthes hyssopoides (L.) Benthem.

Scrophulariaceae

Leaves linear-lanceolate, narrowed to base; palmately nerved: Pedicel up to 4 cm. long. Corolla over 1 cm. long, white tinged with bluish-purple. stamens 2; staminodes 2, glandular, clavate. Capsule elongated, deflexed.

August to March.

India, Sri Lanka. Very common in marshy, harvested rice-fields across plains, Karnataka.

26.6 **Lindernia ruellioides (Colsm.) Penn.**

Bonnaya reptans (Roxb.) Spr.

Gratiola reptans Roxb.

G. ruellioides Colsm.

Scrophulariaceae

Erect, simple or branched, glabrous, annual herbs. Stems creeping and rooting at the base. Leaves on 0.2-0.25 cm. long petioles, ovate-oblong, acute and often decurrent at base, obtuse or rounded at apex, 0.7-3 x 0.4-2 cm. Flowers in glabrous raoemes. Bracts subulate, 0.2-0.5 cm. long. Pedicels 0.5-1 cm. long. Calyx 0.5-0.6 cm. long, glabrous; Segments linear-lanceolate. Corolla bluish purple, 1-1.5 cm. long. Fertile stamens 2. staminodes clavate. capsule cylindrical, 1-1.5 cm. long.

September to November

Siwaliks in Uttar Pradesh, common in rice fields.

20.7 **Bonnaya veronicaefolia** Spreng.

Decumbent or creeping herb. Stem 4-sided; branches ascending, often rooting at the modes. Leaves 1/2-1 in. about long, oblong or oblong-lanceolate or obovate, rather distantly serrate or the lower sometimes subentire. Flowers in terminal and axillary racemes. Calyx deeply divided, segments linear lanceolate, acute. Corolla 1/4-1/8 in. long, violet streaked with purple. Capsules slender, erect or some what spreading, about twice as long as the calyx.

Throughout India and in Ceylon. Western Himalaya up to 5,000 ft. extending to Malaya Peninsula and Islands, Siem, China and the Philippines. Very common all over the area under Upper Gangetic Plains and Siwaliks and adjacent Himalayan sub-tracts.

20.8 **Vandelia hirsuta** Benth.

Scrophulariaceae

Erect succulent herb. Leaves alternate, 2-3 by .5-7 in. (in specific plants), oblanceolate, decurrent, entire or crenate. Flowers in simple densely woolly spike. Calyx segments 5. Corolla rotate; lobes 5. Staments 5, fertile; 2 glabrous, 3 hairy. Capsule septicidal; seeds winged.

September or around.

Assam, Aka hills.

20.9 Bonnaya reptans Spreng. syn. *Hybanthes ciliata* (Colsm.) O. Ktze. Sam-thang-lang, Sam-gichhok (Gare); Kauridarya (Lakimpur).

Weed or roadside trailing herb. Leaves opposite, .5-2 in. by .3-.8 in., ovate-oblong, sharply serrate; petiole. .1-.5 in. long. Flowers in racemes; pedicels short, oblanceolate. Corolla purplish, .75 in. long. Capsule very slender, about 1 in. long, much longer than the calyx.

October to March.

Assam Province, Garo hills, Lakhimpur.

20.10 Bonnaya brachiata Link & Otte. syn. *Gratiola serrata* Roxb. Small rigid glabrous herb, 3-10 in. high. stem 4-sided, the lowest branches decumbent below. Leaves sessile, upto 1 in. long, oblong, obtuse or subacute, closely and deeply spinose-serrate, glabrous. Flowers shortly padicelled, forming terminal racemes; pedicels about equalling the calyx, rigid; bracts lanceolate, lowermost often dentate. calyx about 1/8 in long deeply divided; segments narrow, aristate. Corolla 1/4 in. long, pink or white. Staminodes short, pubescent. Capsules 1/4 in. long, narrowly cylndric, diverging, acute, glabrous. seeds minute, usually tuncate at both ends.

Rainy season.

Throughout India and in Ceylon; Himalayas up to 5,000 ft. extending to the Malay Peninsula, Java, China and the Phillippines. Plant abundant within the areas of Upper Gangetic Plains, Siwalks and sub-Himalayan tracts.

20.11 **Lindernia ciliata** (Colsm.) Pennel.

Gratiola ciliata Colsm.

G. serrata Roxb.

Hybanthes serrata (Roxb.) Urban,

Scrophulariaceae

Herb. Leaves sessile, oblong, penninerved, up to 2.5 x 0.5 cm.; serratous articulate. Flowers in terminal racemes. Carolla pinkish-white. Stamens 3 2; staminodes 2. capsule more than twice the length of calyx.

August to November.

Indomalayisa. Occasional in western plains and lower Ghats, Karnataka state; Southern region, India.

20.12 Lindernia ciliats (Colsm.) Penn. Syns. *Gratiela ciliate* Colsm *Bennaya brachiata* Link & Otte.

Eerct, simple or bnched from the base, annual herbs, 3-20 cm. tall. Stems often decumbent and rooting at base, 4-angular glabrous except-hirsute angles. Leaves sessile, lanceelateoblang or obovate, obtuse or rounded, nearly glabrous, acutely densely serrate with bristle-tipped teeth, 1-3 x 0.5.5-1 cm. Flowers in 3 to 15-flowered racemes. Bracts linear, 0.3-0.5 cm. long. Pedicels widely patent, 0.25-0.5 cm. long. Calyx 0.5cm long, keeled, segments linear-lanceolate, finely acuminate, ciliate. Corolla white with red streaks and dots 0.5-0.8 cm. long. Fertile stamens 2. Capsule cylindric, linear 0.7-0.8 (-1) cm. long.

20.13 Some other species of *Lindernia* Ail. may be referred as few of them are also medicinally useful :

Lindernia oppositifolia 'Retz.) Muk.

Lindernnia crustacea (L.) F. Mueller

Capraria crustacea L.

Vandellia crustacea (L.) Bentham.

Lindernia nummulariifolia (D. Den.) Wettstein. ('Hummularifolia')

Vandellia nummularifolia D. Don.

V. sessiliflora Bentham.

Lindernia parviflora (Roxb.) Haines.

Gratiola parviflora Roxb.

Hybanthes parviflora (Roxb.) Bentham.

Lindernia pusilla Willd.) Boldingh.

Gratiola pusilla Willd.

Selago pusilla Thub.

Torenia hirta Cham. & Schl.

Vandelia scabra Benth.

Lindernia hirta (C. & S.) Pennel.

Lindernia multiflora (Roxb.) Mukerjee.

Torenia multiflora Roxb.

Vandellia multiflora (Roxb.) G. Don.

Lindernia sessiliflora (Renth.) Wettst.

Vandellia sessiliflora Benth.

Lindernia viscosa (Rornom.) Morr.

Gratiola viscosa Hornem.

Vandellia hirsuta Roxb.

Lindernia hirsuta (Benth.) Wetst.

20.14 Lindernia Allioni is sometimes segregated into *Vandellia* Linn., *Bonnaya* Link & Otte, *Hybanthes* Rafin. and *Lindernia Lindernia crustacea* (Linn.) F. Muell is variable in habit, size and shape of leaves, size of flowers and capsules, Biosystematic observations may understand the pattern of variation in this polymorphic taxon.

Lindernia nummularifolia (D. Den.) Wettst. is closely allied to *L. sessiliflora* (Benth.) Wettst., but this is easily recognizable by distinctly pedicelled flowers, longer calyx, corolla and capsules; whereas *L. sersiliflora* (Benth.) Wettst is very closely allied (indeed reduced) to *L. nummularifolia* (D. Den.) wettst., and distinguishable by sessile flowers, longer calyx, and corolla, and long-acuminate capsules. Further observations may elucidate the interrelationships between these two not distantly related taxa.

The plants are chasmogamous with pedicelled, pink flowers in summers and during the heavy monsoons they are cleistegamous with tiny, white, sessile flowers and clusters of sessile capsules (somtimes both types of flowers found on same plant). the chasmogamous form is named *Lindernia nummulariifolia* and the cleistagamous form is *L. sessiliflora. Lindernia* All. in general is taxonomically interesting for different aspects involving various species and genera in relevance.

Lindernia parviflora (Roxb.) Haines. is closely allied to *L. prrcumbens* (krock.) Phileox. (*L. pyxidaria all.)* but this is easily reconizable by 3-nerved leaves, 2 fertile stamens and elliptic capsules longer than the calyx; as *L. precumbens* (Krock.) Phileox. is radily distinguishable from *L. parviflora* (Roxb.) Hanies. (often confusing) by 3 to 5 nerved, 4 fertile stamens, absence of staminodes and ovoid capsules as long as the clayx.

20.15 Various species of *Lindernia* All. are medicinally useful, and also used in veterniary medicine.

The leaves of *Lindernia anagallia* (Burm. f.) Pennell. are mde into a paste and applied in headache.

The plant *Lindernia antipods* (L.) Alston. Syn. *Bennaya veronicaefolia* Spreng. is useful in abdominal pain, cholera, convulscence, cough, delirium, dysuria, night fever, ringworm, small-pox, snake-bite and syphilis.

The leaves of *Lindernia oppositifolia* (Retz.) Muk. are useful to prevent miscarriage. Plant is called panchamanl. *Lindernia ruelloides* (Colsm.) pennel. syn. *Bonnaya reptans* (Roxb.) Spr. is medicinally used. Leaves are useful in urinary complaints.

The plants of *Lindernia hyssopioides* (L.) Haines are also used in veterinary medicine. Leaves are employed to remove parasitic insects in cattles. The whole herb of *Bonnaya reptans* Spreng. is applied externally for worms in the skin.

The plant of *Vandelia pyxidaria* Maxim. is used in ghrita as a remedy for gonorrhoea.

Juice of the here is given to children ins cases of diarrhoea specially affected with green stool.

The plant of *V. pedunculata Benth.* is medicinally used for the purposes as *V. pyxidaria* Maxim.

21. BHĀRATI-ṚJUKAṆṬĀ-KṚṢṆASATINAPHA-LĀSITĀHARITAPUṢPĀ-RAKTOŚODHIKĀ

M21. Maytenus senagalensis (Lamk.) Exell.

Maytenus emarginata (Willd.) Ding-Hu.

M. senagalensis Lamk.

Celastrus emarginatus Wills.

C. montana Roth.

Gymnosporia montana (Roth.) Bentham.

G. emarginata (Willd.) Thwaites.

Celastraceae

Dantiya-cettu, Henkol, Kentei, Vice; Vingar (Baluchistan), Baikal (Hindi), Kakra (Rajsthan), Bharati (Marathi), Danti (Telagu), Tundrasi (Kannara).

Tall spinous shrub or small tree, with stiff branches forming a loose crown, glabrous glaucous of pale green; spines straight, axillary, 1-2 in. long and often bearing leaves and flowers. Leaves obovate to linear-spathulate, but very variable in form and size, entire or crenate, coraceeus. Cymes axillary and shorter than the leaves, or on the spines, rigid, divaricating. Flowers small, greenish-white, often sterile. Bracts, calyx-lobes and petiole fimbriate, Disk broad, flat, 10-lobed. Anthers versatile. stamens lobed. Capsule globose or avoid, black, about the size of a small pea, 1-5-celled. Cells usually 1-seeded. Rainy to spring season; various times throughout the year. Punjab, parasnath in Bihar and drier parts of southern and central India, Siwalik, Merwar, Bundelkhand, Central Africa, Malay Archipelago and Australia.

21.1 Gymnosporia montana Lawson.

Tall shrub or small tree under favourable circumstances, trunk, short, crooked. Leaves grey, coriaceous, exceedingly variable in shape and size, obovate, oblanceolate to linear-spathulate, narrowed into the petile. Flowers small, pale greenish, white, cymes axillary or fasciculate on short branchlets, often forming terminal elongate penicles. capsule 1/2 in., usually 2-valved, seeds 1-2, rarely 3, with or wiithout an arillus.

Common in the Punjab, Sind, Rajputana, Central Provinces, Bihar and drier parts of Peninsula.

21.2 Maytenus emarginatus (Willd.) Ding Hou. Armed or unarmed, erect shrubs. Leaves 4-7 x 2-4 cm., usually obovate and emarginate, serrate, drying a glaucous green or reddish-brown. Inflorescence axillary, extra-axillary or borne at tip of spines, pedunculate, Flower white. Sepals 5, petals 5; capsule usually concave at tip.

Indomalaysia. Common in plains and upper (Ghats, usually in open country or in association in deciduous forests, Karnataka.

21.3 **Gymnosporia rayleana** Wall.

Celastrus spinosa Royle.

Gynosporia royleana Lawson.

Celastraceae

Gwala darim (Dzaral (Trans. Ind.), Pataki, Kander (Punjab), Baikal (Hindi), Vaichigachha (Bengla), Kharai (Punjab), Kattanji (Tamil), Dantausi (Telgu).

Stiff dense shrub 8-12 ft. high. Leaves ovate, acute, greyish, spines axillary, slender. Cymes mostly axillary, petals reddish with white edges. Fruits 1/3 in diam.

Almost throughout the year.

Punjab, Shub-Himalayan tract, east to Kumaon.

21.4 **Gymnosporia royleana** M. Lawson.

Jalidhar (Hindi), Kandiari (Punjabi), Gwaldari (U.P.Hills), Danti (Telgu).

Armed shrub. Western Himalayas, Kumaon and Garhwal upto 4, 5000 ft.

21.5 Gymnosporia spinosa Royle syn. *G. royleana* Lawson. A glabrous densely-branching shrub, armed with stiff straight axillary spines. Leaves shortly stalked 3/4 to 1-3/4 in. long, broadly ovate or obovate, crenate or nearly entire, coriaceous, dull greyish-green. Cymes axillary subsessile, often fascicled on short dichotomous branches. Bracts and calyx-lobes ciliate. Petals oblong, white or reddish with white margins. Stamens inserted under the edge of the disk; anthers versatile. Disk 5-lobed, surrounding the base of the 3-colled ovary. Capsule 1/3 in. long, turbinate, 3-cornered and 3-colled. seeds partialy covered with an aril. Outer Western Himalaya, from the Jumna to Kumann, up to

4,000 ft., also in the Punjab and extending into Afghanistan. Siwalik range, Bundelkhand, Uttar Pradesh.

21.6 **Maytenus rothiana** (Walp.) Ramam.

Celastrus serrulatus Roth.

Catha rothiana Walp.

Gymnosporia rothiana (Walp.) **Lawson.**

Maytenus wighiana Babu

Celastraceae

Unarmed, scandent shrubs up to 3-4 m. height. Leaves 9-10 x 5-6 cm., broadly elliptic-obovate, narrowed and acute at base, obtuse at tip. Flower white. Fruit 5-seeded.

April or summer season.

Shout-western India. Occasional amongst undergrowth of semievergeeen forests in lower Ghats, Karnataka state.

21.7 **Maytenus falconeri** (Lawason) M.A. Rau

Gymnosporia falconeri Lawson.

Celastraceae

Erect evergreen shrub, 10-25 cm. high. Leaves 2-6 cm. long, elliptic or ovate, serrulate, clothed on both surfaces with agort white pubescent which is denser beneath. Flowers small in fascicled axillary few-flowered cymes. Capsule about 1 cm. long, turbinate, 3-colled, slightly lobed, smooth, brown, seeds enclosed in white aril.

March to December

Fairly common throughout the sub-Himalayan tract, Kumaon region, Teral-Bhawar, Uttar Pradesh.

21.8 **Maytenus falconeri** (Lawson) M. A. Ranu var. *Kanjilalli* Raizada Shrub has difference in features from typical *Maytenus falconeri* in having glabrous leaves, smooth, on both surfaces, and longer and larger fruit with size 9 mm-14 mm. long.

Eastern Uttar Pradesh, Upper Gangetic Plains. The shrubs or small trees, differing from *Celastrus* Linn. by flowers in dichotomous cymes and stamens inserted under the disk.

Broadly the species of *Gymnosperia* W. et A. are grouped on spinescent features. They are distinguished by armed, spines often bearing leaves and flowers and armed with spines usually naked. Under armed groups, the western and eastern species are characterized.

21.9 Gymnosporia cuminata Hakk f. A large shrub or small tree. Leaves lanceolate, crenate-serrate, 3-7 in., narrowed into the short petiole. Cymes solitary or fascicled, axillary or on short lateral tubercles, peduncles and pedicels filiform. Capsules 1/3 in. longly, mostly 2-valved, 2-seeded, lower half of seed enclosed in a faciniate arillus. Assam, Khasi hills, Sikkim. Butan, Upper Burma.

Gymnosporia neglecta Lawson. A shrub with leaves elliptic, serrate, blade 4-6, petiole 1/3-1/2 in; fruits globose 1/3 in. long, 3-valved and seeds 1-3. Assam, Khasi hills.

Gymnosporia oblanceolata Lawsen. A shrub with leaves oblanceolate, serrate in the upper half, 3-4 x 3/4 in., tapering into short petiole; sec. n. 5-6 pair very oblique. Irrawadi.

Gymnosporia salicifolia Lawson. A shrub with leaves narrowly lanceolate, serrate, 3-4 x 1/2 in. and sec. n. faint. Assam. province.

21.10 The foregoing eastern species are unarmed and other following unarmed species are western.

Gymnosporia ovata Wall. with leaves 2-2 in. cymes much branched, axillary and terminal, one in. long; flowers about 1/6-1/8 in. across; capsules 1/2 in. diam. Nilgiris, Malabar and Palni hills, southern India.

Gymonsporia rothiana W. et A. A small tree, with leaves obovate, narrowed into petiole 3 in. long; cymes dense, nearly sessile, mostly below the leaves; fruits obovoid 1/2-3/4 in long. Plant sometimes armed.

Gymnosporia puberula Lawson. Inflorescence and undersides of leaves slightly pubescent; leaves membranous, obovate, acute, 2-3 in. long, narrowed into short petiole; cymes lax, few-fid, peduncles and pedicels filiform. Konkan,

21.11 Two species of *Maytenus* Molina are diatinguished. *Maytenus emarginata* (Willd.) Ding Hou is armed or unarmed, erect and deciduous shrubs with crenulate leaves and flowers in cymes and peduncled; whereas *Maytenus rothiana* (Walp.) Raman. is unarmed, scandent and evergreen shrub with leaves entire and flowers fascicled and sessile.

Gymnosporia Benth. & Hook. F. is merged with *Maytenus* Molina. Erect spinous shrubs, flowers in axillary cymes, stamens inserted beneath the margin of the disk of two relevant species of *Celastrus* Linn. which are separated by capsules characters, as the capsule turbinate and 3-cornered in *C. spinos* a Royle and capsule globose in *C. senegalensis* Lamk. in genral *Celastrus* Linn. and *Maytenus* Molina are with alternate leaves (when various others have opposite leayes); and *Maytenus* Mol. plants are usually armed erect or scandent shrubs, when *Celastrus* Linn. Plants are unarmed shrubby climbers, with other characteristic differences in various species.

21.12 Various species of ***Maytenus*** Mol. are medicinally useful. The smoke from the seeds of *Gymnosporia* M. Law. is considered helpful to relieve toothache. The bark of *Gymnosperia spinosa* (Forsk.) Fiori is ground to a paste applied with mustard oil to destroy padiculi. The fruits of *Maytenus senegalensis* (Lamk.) Exell. Syn. *M. emarginata* (Willd.) Ding-Hu. are useful as blood purifier. Leaves are useful in cough. Leaves are considered useful in eye complaints. Fruits are edible.

Plant is also useful in veterinary medicine. Roots are used as rejuvenator medicine.

Twigs of plant are signified for religious ceremonies.

22. ŚALKABAHULĀ-VṚNTAPATRĀ-RAKTĀNILAPUṢPĪ-NIRJHARĀSANNĀ-ROPAṆIKĀ

M22. Melastema malabathricum Linn.

Melastema malabathricum Linn.(*'malabathrica'*)

incl. *M. normale* Den.)

Melastemaceae

Futki (Assamese), Myetpye (Lower Burma), Shame (Upper Burma), Mystype (Burmese), Kodalai (Tamil), Pattude (Telugu), Kotali (Malayalam), Palore (Marathi), Karoti (Uriya); Futiki, Jatrangi, Pudiralu, Useh-Kathlew.

Evergreen shrub or small tree, branchlets, petioles and peduncles densely clothed with acute or acuminate, often serrulate scales. Leaves 3-5-nerved, strigose and often tomentose on the underside, blade 2-6, petiole up to about 1/2 in. long. Flowers purple, 2-3 in. across, calyx densely clothed with pale linear acuminate entire or serrate scales. Fruit 1/4 in. diam.

Different seasons; throughout the year, chiefly March-July. Sub-Himalayan tract and outer hills from Nepal eastwards, ascending in Sikkim to 6, 000 ft. elevation; Assam, Khasi hills, chittagong, Andamans, Burma, Western Peninusula.

22.1 **Melastoma malabathricum Linn.**

Shrub. Leaves 8-15 X 3.5-6 cm. elliptic-lanceelate, acute at both ends, triplinerved scaly. Calyx lobes deciduous. Petals large, showy, broadly obovate, purplish. Larger stamens purple, smaller ones yellow.

India; common in wet deciduous to semi-evergreen forests in Ghats, near brooks and streams, Karnataka; Southern regions in country.

Ccylon moist country to 8,000 ft. elevation, Seyebelles, Malay Peninsula and Archipelago. China, Australia, New Calesdonia and countries.

22.2 **Melastema decemfidum** Roxb.

Melastema sanguineum Sima.

Melastemaceae

Shrub. Branchlets, petioles and peduncles clothed with long spreading bristles. Leaves scattered, appressed hairs.

Burma, Malay peninsula, Cochin-China, Tenasserim, Malaya, Tokin, China.

22.3 Some other allied species of *Melastema* Linn. may also be referred;

Melastoma imbricatum Wall.

Shrub. Branchlets, petioles, peduncles and calyx clothed with closely appressed serrulate scales. Leaves strigose on both sides, appressed scales on nerves beneath, blade 4-9, petiole 1/2 to 1.5 in. long. Flowers 1/1.4 in across petals oblong.

Assam, Khasi hills, Andmans, Burma.

22.4 **Melastema clarkaenum** Cegniaux.

Melastema houtteanum (Kurz. (Not Naudin)

Shrub. Calyx-tube clothed with ciliate pale coloured scales about 1/6 in. long.

Pegu, Burma, Tenasserim.

22.5 The species of *Melastoma* Linn. are medicinally useful and employed in allied purposes.

The roots of *Melastoma malabathricum* Linn. syn. *Melastoma normale* L. are used in blood dysentery. Leaves are ground and applied to cuts and bruises. Leaves are considered useful in diarrhoea. Leaves are suggested to be useful as haemostatic remedy.

The leaves of plant and also roots are considered useful in small pox.

Leaves and roots are externally applied over wounds and ulcers.

Fruits are edible.

23. MONATARU-MĀMSAPHALA-TRIKAṆṬAKĀ-HARITAPRASAVĀ-KALARAKṢIK

M23. Meyna laxifilora Robyns.

Vangueria spinosa Hook. F.

V. pubescens Kurz.

V. edulis Miq.

V. mollis Wall.

Rubiaceae

Muyuna, Myuna, Muduna, Mainphal, Mainakatan (Hindi and Bengla), Alu, Hulee, Halawani, (Marathi), Alu (Gujrati), Cegagadda (Telgu), Veliki, Visikilema (Telgu), Nanakkarai (Tamil), Mullakare (Kannarese), Gundkare, Gebergally (Kan), Gurbeli, Meltakanta (Oriya); Biobindi, Ketkora, Thiksing, Dieng-soh-men; Ketkora, Mon (Assam)

Small tree or large bush, with straight opposite simple or 3-nate spines. Leaves 3-4 in., opposite or 3-nately whorled, ovate or oblong, acute or acuminate; petiole half to one inch; stipule cuspidate from a broad base. cymes 1-1.5 in., shortly peduncled; flowers greenish, pedicelled. Calyx 5-toothed. Corolla-tibe sub-globose; lobes triangular, acute. Style glabrous; stigma 4-5 lobed.

Drupe about 2/4 in. diam., subglobose or turbinate, smooth, fleshy; pyrenes 4-5, woody, smooth.

Cold to rainy seasons. Java, from northern Bengal to Canara, Pegu, Tenasserim, Burma.

23.1 Vangueria spinosa Roxb.

Spinescent small tree, therny. Leaves membranous, ovate or evate-lanceolate, glabrous or tementose, blade 3-5, petole half inch long, Stipules early deciduous. Flowers pentamerous, greenish, calyx-segments from s triangular base linear, nearly as long as the 5-celled ovary, corolla-lobes acuminate, Drupe yellow half to 1 inch in diam., fleshy, with 4-5 smooth hard 1- seeded stones.

Sikkim Terai, along roadsides, Jowal, Khasi hills, Lower Bengal, Burma, Upper and Lower, deciduous forests of the Peninsula.

23.2 Meyna laxiflora Robyns syn. *Vangueria spinosa* Roxb. Thrrny, small trees. Leaves elliptic-lanceelate, acuminate, up to 12 x 6 cm. cyme short, lax. Pedicels up to 3 cm. Corolla greenish-white. Drupe ellipseid, 2 cm across, dry. Indomalaysia. Occasional in Upper Ghats, Karnataka state.

23.3 Meyna laxiflora Robyns. syn. *Vangueria spinosa* Hock. f. (in part) A spinescent or unarmed shrub or small tree found in western Uttar Pradesh, Bengal, Assam and the Deccan Peninsula; with leaves ovate to elliptic; flowers in lax cymes, greenish white, drupes sub-globose, c. 2.5 cm. diam., smooth, green to brown, succulent; seeds albuminous, with a mebranous testa.

23.4 **Vangueria spinosa** Roxb.

Thichkeeng (Gare), Men (Cah.), Misthei (Kuki), Haibi (Manipur) Seh-men, Dieng-seh-myren (Khasi), Dieng-sa-matan (Sylhet), Mon, Ketkora (Assam). Deciduous shrub or small tree. Bark brown to deep grey with vertical cracks; blaze yellowish. Spines up to .7 in. long, somewhat supra-axillary; branchlets terete. Leaves opposite or sometimes ternate, 1.5-5 by 1.2.75 in., entire, ovate elliptic or elliptic-ovate, acute or bluntly acuminate, membranous, more or less glabrous; lateral nerves 0.9 on either half, curving upwards near the margin; nerve axils with tufts of hair; base shortly cuneate; petiole. 2-5. in. long; stipules connate, cuspidate from a brown base. Flowers greenish white, on short peduncled cymes, which are axillary or supra-axillary or sometimes frim small excerscences. Calyx 5-toothed. Corolla induplicate-valvate in bud; tube short, sub-globose; throat woolly; lobes spreading. Stamens sub-sessile; anthers exserted. Ovary 5-colled, less often 3-4 celled or 6 celled; style long; stigmas lobed; ovules pendulous, solitary. Fruit a fleshy drupes; about 1-1.5 in.across, yellowish when ripe, with 3-5 woody pyrenes; embryo central in copious fleshy albumen.

Summers to rainy season; April to September.

Assam prevince, Gare hills, Sibsagar, K. & I. Hills, N.E. Frontiers Tract, Kamrup, Cachar, Darrang and Golpara.

23.4 Meyna laxiflora Robyns. Syn. *V. spinosa* sensu Hook. f.; *Meyna pubescens* (Kurz.) Robyns. Syns. *V. pubescens* Kurz. *V.*, *spinosa* auct. non. Roxb. *V. spinosa* var *Mollis* wall ex Hook. f, Meyna spinosa Royli ex link. Syn *V. spinosa* Roxb. are treated three species.

23.5 The plant *Meyna laxiflora* Robyns. syn. *Vangueria spinosa* Hook. is medicinally useful and has allied usses.

The dry fruit is considered narcetic and it is useful for boils and dysentery. The powdered leaves are said to be good for diptheria.

The fruits are edible. Leaves are pounded and eaten. Leaves are also used as fodder, but are of a poor quality.

The decorticated seeds on extraction with benzene yileds 38.5% fat; and the component fatty acids of the oil are palmitic, stearic, oleic and linoleic oils.

Fruits are cooling, refrigerant, cholagogue, strengthening and an expellant of phlegm and bile. Powdered leaves are useful in diptheria

The roots of *Meyna laxiflora* Robins. are useful in abdominal pain and colic. Leaves are useful in dysentery. Plants is useful in fissures in skin. It is used in dipthaeria. Fruits are edible.

The leaves of *Meyna spinesa* syne. *M. pubescens* Robins. and *Vangueria spinosa* Roxb. are useful in diptheria and dysentery. Leaves are edible, and useful as salad and vegetable.

24. SĀKANĀRI̤-REKHITKĀṆḌĀ-RODHĀSRIKĀ-ĀNTRASUKH-DHAVALAPRASAVĀ

M24. **Mikania cordata** (Burm. f.) Robinson.

Eupatorium cordatum Burma f.

Mikania scandens (auct. non Willd) Clarke.

Asteraceas

German-pula, Nari, Japan-za, Momosha. Thap, Ranusinga.

Twining herb; stem angular, striate, twisted, puberulous. Leaves 2-9-7 cm. long, 2-4 cm, broad, ovate, opposite, crenate along margins, glabrous, acute or acuminate at apex, cordate, hastate or rarely truncite at base, petioles 1-5.5 cm.long. Heads 3.5-6 cm. long, 2.2-0.5 cm. across, 4-flowered, homogamous, in paniculate, corymbose clusters terminating lateral branches; branchlets angled; peduncles absent or up to 2-4 mm. long, slender, involucre oblong-tubular bracts 4, 1-seriate, each 3.5-4 mm. long, narrowly oblong-obovate; glabrous, acuminate at apex, receptacle small, flat, naked. Flowers all tubular, hermaphrodite, regular, white, regular, white, fertile, corolla about 3 mm. long, regular; tube slender, limb campanulate, 5-lobed, lobes acute, sparsely hairy without. Anthers appendiculate at apex, obtuse at base. Style thick, glabrous, style-arms about 2.5 mm. long, flattened, minutely papillate, acute at apex. Cypsela abou 1.5 mm, long, linear-oblong, 4-angled, minutely glandular, black or blackish-brown, truncate at apex. Pappus 2.75-3 mm. long, numerous, 1-seriate, scaberulous, white, sometime pale purplish in fruit, connate at base in a ring.

November to February.

Assam, Bengal, Tripura, Sikkim Eastern India Assam region; Bhutan, Neraha in Southern India.

Burma, Malaya Peninsula, Indo-China, East Indies, Siam, Formesa, Philippines, Central and North America.

24.1 **Chromolaena odorata** (L.) King. & Robinson.

Eupatorium odoratum L.

Asteraceae

Assam Deta (Assamese);

Gandhuri., Kotojora, Rukusi, Kusuri, Kengiurungion, Krahlynroh, Phulgandhuri, Samsimari, Telimbabe, Zaman, Zemlu.

Undershrub. Leaves up to 10 x 5 cm., ovate to rhomboid, acute, crenate-serrate, subpalmately 3-nerved, Corolla white to purple

November to April.

Adventive Neotropical weed. A spreading weed in Ghats (Assan), Karnataka state, in southern India.

24.2 Eupatorium odoratum Linn. syn. E. cenyzoides Mill., *E. conyzoides* Vahl.

Erect or scrambling perennial herbs. Stems often much-branched from the base, often decumbent below, glandular pubescent. Leaves one 1-2 cm. long petiole, ovate-lanceolate or triangular, acute or acuminate, cuneate at base, entire or serrsto-dentate, nearly glabrous, gland-punctate on the lower surface, 2-10 k. 0.5-3 cm. Heada in terminal corymbs, 0.3-0.4 cm. across. 1 cm. long. Involucral bracts 3 to 4 (-5) - seriate, ovate-lanceolate, sharply acute, 0.1-0.7 cm. long. Corolla pale violet 0.5 cm. long. Achenes 5-angular, glabrous, 0.4 cm. long. Pappus-hairs whitish, 0.5 cm. long.

September to November.

Siwalik region (Dehradun) in Uttar Pradesh; cultivated, rarely mot wth as an escape in waste places.

24.3 **Eupatoruum cannabinum** Linn.

Asteraceae

Samsing, Durasammok (Gare); Tongel-lati (Assamese), Samkhabli Kachar), Long-renchick (Kuki), Kembat-mang-rim (Khasi), Kal-bun (Mikyang).

Coarse perennial, often straggling. Leaves. 8-4.5 by .3-2.5 in., usually opposite sometimes alternate, lanceolate, ovate-lanceolate. coarsly serrate, acuminate, scabrid above, pubescent beneath, lateral nerves almost obscure; base narrowed into the petiole; petiole up to .7 in. long. flowers heads corymbose, homogenous. Involucral-bracts oblong, many seriate, unequal, ribbed or channeled; outer ones shorter; receptacle naked. Corolla regular, tubular, 5-bobed. Stamens syngenesious; anther appendaged. style-arms long, obtuse. Fruit truncate, black with 5 ridges. Pappus white, filiform, 1-seriate, numerous, rigid, about twice the length of the fruit.

November to December, cold season.

Assam prvinces; Darrang, Kamrup, Gare Hills, North Cachar Hill,s Khasi and Jaintia Hills.

24.4 **Eupatorium adenophorum** Spreng.

Eupatorium glandulosum HBK.

Ageratina adenophora (Spreng.) King. & Rob.

Asteraceae

Azatesen (Langsec, Nhasa, Panasri, Poekiduva.

Straggling, perrennial branched undershrub. Branches cylindrical reddish, densely glandular hairy. beaves apposite, petioled, rhomboid-ovaid, trapezoid or almost angular; sharply pointed, coarsely serrate above the cuneate base, 2.5-9 cm. long, nearly glabrous above, hispidulous along the nerves and glabrous (glabrate) beneath, obscurely glandular on the petiole which is 2.5-cm. long. and on lower surfaces corymbs fastigate-trichotomous, flowerheads clustered, white, pedicelled, 40-70 flowered, slightly fragrant; receptacles flat; involucral bracts, about twenty in two rows, lanceolate, acuminate, striate, glandular-ciliate, mostly subequal shorter than than the florets, with scarious margins and with two well-defined nerves. Corolla-tubes white, 1mm.slender, abruptly dilated. Style-arms long and far exserted, divergent. Achenes bkack, glabrous, slender, crowned by a pappus of 10-12 white scabrid hairs, twice as long.

March to July.

Introduced and later naturalised in India. Native of Mexico and Jamaica.

24.5 **Eupatorium adenophorum** Spreng.

Erect, widely branched, somewhat foetid, annual-perennial herbs, often with a woody base. Stems dark purple, gland-hairy. Leaves with 3-4 cm. long, gland-hairy petioles, ovate or ovate-rhomboid, with a truncate or cuneate base, acute or acuminate, crenate-serrate, glabrous except hairy nerves beneath. Heads in axillary and terminal, gland-hairy corymbs combined, 3 serate, linear-lanceolate, acute, 0.6-0.7 cm. across, short-peduncled, Involucral bracts 3-seriate, linear-lanceolate, acute, gland-hairy, 0.3-0.5 cm. long. Corolla white, 0.25-0.3 cm. long. Achenes 5-angular, glabrous, black, 0.2 cm. long. Pappus-hairs whitish, 0.35 cm. long.

Common in ravine slopes and grassy localities in Siwalik region (Dehradun) in Uttar Pradesh. Native of Central America, Naturalised.

Initially plant introduced as garden herb and afterwards running wild and later naturalised in different regions. Falry common in Chir plantations, common along streams and other localities in northern region particularly in the Siwaliks zone and also in other areas.

24.6 Three species of *Eupatorium* Linn. are distinguishable. Involucral bracts 1 to 2-seriate and the achenes hairy on the ribs in *Eupatorium riparium* Regal. ; whereas other two species are with involucral bracts 3 to 5-seriate and the achenes glabrous, and they arr further distinguished. Stems, petioles and imvolucral bracts gland-hairy, and corolla white in *Eupatorium adenophorum Linn; when E. odoratum Linn. is* with corolla light violet but gland-hairs absent.

Eupatorium conyzoides Mill. and *E. conyzoides* Vahl. are conspecific with *E. odoratm* Linn (hitherto considered distinct species) which is present name of the plant *Eupatorium odoratum* Linn.

The plant *Mikania cordata* (Burm. f.) Robinson is common in waste places, on hedges and bushes in shady situations and twining on *Diospyros montana* and *Cordia dictotoma* in various areas in Uttar Pradesh (Aligarh district).

Mikania micrantha Kunth. is synonymous to *M. scandens* auct. non Willd. and *M. cordata* var. *indica* Kitamura Loose aggregate of *Mikania scandens* is suggested into different species. The Old World plants are referable to the species *Mikania cordata* (Burm. f.) Robinson, since they have difference from *Mikania scandens* wild. of North America in their open inflorescence slightly larger heads, more pointed involucral bracts and numerous pappus. Recently the species most common in the Indian region is *Mikania micrantha* HBK., a species of South American origin and well known in West Indies and not *Mikania cordata* or *M. scandens* which are supposed to be prevalent in Eastern India. Hence, the species of *Mikania*, common in Eastern India, Pakistan appears to be *N. micrantha* HBK.

24.7 Various species relevant is *Mikania, Eupatorium* and *Chromolaena* are medicinally useful.

The stems of *Mikania Micrantha* H.B.K. syns. *M. cordata* (surm. f.) Robinson, *M. scandens* Willd. are useful in condition of constipation and indigestion. Leaves of the plants are pounded and applied over wounds and cuts. Leaves are also useful in injuries and bleeding wounds.

The leaves are considered effective as haemostatic and used in various ailing conditions for haemostatic properties.

Leaves of herb are useful in dysentery and diarrhoea including bleeding dysentery and gripping. It is also helpful to check indigestion and regularise bowels. Leaves after grinding or their juice may be suggested for use in the conditions. Leaves are similarly considered useful in stomach troubles. Leaves are generally, considered useful in gastrointestinal disorders, or favourable to disestion, as the leaves are edible and used as vegetable.

Leaves are useful in headache, and some others ailments. Similarly the stems are considered useful.

Whole plant of *Mikania scandens* Wild. is considered as useful remedy being antidote to snake bite as well as scorpion sting.

Mikania micrantha H.B.K. syn. *M. scandens* willd. is known by various names such as German-Pula, Japan-za, Monoshathap, Mari, Rangusinga, and the plant is utilised as medicinal herb and also as a edible plant, in different parts of various regions.

Plant has importance in biological activity as an anti-amphetamine phytoagents.

Plant of *Eupatorium odoratum* Linn. is considered a fish poison and used for this purpose.

The herb of *Eupatorum canabinum* Linn. is medicinally potrnt and used in various ailments.

Herb is diaphoretic, duretic, antiscorbutic, cathatic, emetic and antipyretic, and the plant is used in various ailments for the medicinal properties and activity.

Plant is used in jaundice, scurvy and useful for fomenting sores and ulcers including infammation.

Herb is considered useful as emmenagogue and useful in menstrual troubles in female patients. Plants is used as purgative in constipation and other ailing conditions.

The plant contains a bitter substance, eupatorin, inulin and a resin.

It contains euparin, eupatoriopietin etc., and Triterpene tetrarasterol, la-lactucerol, isolation of rutin 10-4%); saponin from leaves. Euporin highest yield up to 0.34% found in cultivated plants.

The plant of *Mikania cordata* (Burm.) B.L. Robinson syn. *M. scandens* Hook. f. (non Willd) is rich source of Vitamins A and C; is also contains vitamin B. Leaves are used against itches and employed for poulticing wounds and boils.

The plant of *Eupatorium cannabinum* Linn. is recommended as a deobstruent in visceral obstruction consequent to intermittent fevers and externally as a discutient in hydrophobic swellings of the legs and scrotum.

The plant *Ageratina adenophora* (Spreng) King. & Robinson syn. *Eupatorium adenophora* Spreng, *E. glandulosum* HBK. is medicinally useful and used in various ailments, as the plant has certain medicinal activities.

Leaves are gound and externally applied to wounds, ulcers, cuts and injuries; and herb especially leaves is used as a haemostatic medicine.

Leaves are used in stomach troubles and the plant is stomachic and useful in stomachache.

Leaves are also useful in toothache and tooth troubles.

The plant *Chromolaena odorata* (Linn). King. & Robinson. syn. *Eupatorium odorata* LInn. are medicinally useful in various ailments by employing its different parts.

Whole plant is useful in bone fractures, and the herb is ground and paste applied over fracture part of body. Other measures of bandazes, splinters and allied are also followed.

Roots are pounded finely and applied externally over the burns lesions. The juice of plant esp. roots is also useful burn cases.

Leaves are roots are topically applied to cuts. Whole plant is ground and applied to sprains and injuries and bruises. Roots are useful in gastric troubles. Leaves are useful in pains. Leaves are given in dysentery. Leaves are also used to stop leeding.

Plant is bait for fish, and poison for earthworns.

25. CĀTURVALLĪ-AṆUPUṢPIKĀ-MĀRĪTASĀKH-KUSUMAPITIKĀ-NĀḌĪBALYĀ

M25. **Myxopyrum serrutulum** A. W. Hill

Myxopyrum smilacifolium C.B. Clarke. (in part, non Blume)

Oleaceae

Chathuravalli (Nalayalam), Chathuramulla, Chathuramulliki (Malayalam), Gohera-lata (Assam)

Large evergreen scandent shrub. branches 4-angular, glabrous. Leaves opposite, oblong to ovate, acuminate, entire, mintuely toothed, coriaceous, 3-nerved or almost 5-nerved, veins reticulated; base cuneate or rounded, often unequal; petiole up to .5 in. long. Flowers minute, yellowish in simple axillary or terminal trichotomous panicles. Calyx urceolate, sharply 4-segmented. Corolla lobes 4, concave, indulplicate valvate in bud, tube longer than the calyx. Stamens 2 on the corolla tube; filaments short; anthers ovate, thick. Ovary 2-celled; stigma nearly sessile, 2-lobed; ovules 1-2 in each cell, attached near the base at the inner angle. Fruit .3 in across, 1-seeded subglobose or 2-seeded; obovoid; pericarp crustaceous, purplish; albumen hairy; radicle inferior.

Cold season.

South Deccan Peninsula and Anamali Mts; Sikkim Terai, Chittagong. Assam province, Mikir Hills, N.E. Frontier Tract, Lakhimpur, Sibsagar, Darrang, Kaumrup, Goalpara, Sylhet, Cachar, N.E. and Gare Hills.

25.1 Myxopyrum smilacifolium Blume

Ligustrum lauriforium Roxb.

Chionanthes smilacifolia Wall.

C. coriaceum wall.

Asteraceae

Nearly glabrous large scandent shrub. Leaves ovate to oblong acute entire or toothed, 6-9 in., from narrow-oblong to cordate-ovate, acuminate, base cuneate or rounded, entire slightly toothed or closely serrate on the same branch; petiole 1/2 in. Panicles 4-8 in., peduncled; branches somewhat lax in fruit.

Malaya, Admiralty Islands, Pegu, Penang. Sikkim, Assam, North-eastern Hills, Bengladesh. Southern India.

25.2 Myxopyrum nervosum Blume.

Oleaceae

Large scandent shrub. Leaves oblong or elliptic acute entire or toothed, 1vs. 8 by 2.5 in. base cuneate or rounded, very coriaceous. Panicles minutely pubescent in flower, very rigid. brachiate in fruit.

Sumatra, Java, Malacca.

25.3 **Myxopyran smilacifolium** C.S. Clarke, A. large twining glabrous evergreen shrub, branches green, more or less quadrangular. Leaves coriaceous, elliptic, entire or serrate, 6-9 pet., numerous in axillary and terminal trichotomous petioles, calyx deeply, 4-cleft, corolla-tube longer than calyx. Fruit half inch in diam., dark purple, in large hanging branches, pericarp crustaceous.

Terai tange of Sikkim Himalayas, North-eastern region, Eastern India, Assam. Burma, Tenasserim.

25.4 **Myxopyrum serrutulum** A.W. Hill.

A large scandent shrub found in western ghats in Wynaad and Travancore at altitudes of 600-900 m. Leaves obovate-elliptic, serrulate; flowers yellow, in axillary or terminal panicles; fruit obovoid with one or two seeds.

25.5 The plan *Myxopyrum serrutulum* A.W. Hill is medicinally useful.

Leaves are useful in respiratory diseases, and rheumatic and nervous complaints.

The leaves are powdered and taken with ghee as a remedy for asthma, cough, rheumatism, nervous complaints and consumption. Leaves ground and boiled in oil are applied in fever, headache, ear diseases and back ache.

26. TORANAVALLĪ-ROMILAŚĀKHI-AVAKARṆIKĀ-SUMĀDHIPATRĀ-GRĀHIKĀ

P26. **Paracalyx scariosa** (Rexb.) All.

Cylista scariosa Roxb.

Fabaceae (Papilionacoae)

Ranghevada (Narathi), Karuchikuda (Talugu); Simbi, Sogurmottu, Teranvel.

Woody climber with slender hairy-downy branches. Leaflets minutely stipellate, 2-4 in., long, ovate or subrhomboidal, acute, subcoriaceous, thinly grey-downy above, densely so below. Flowers in large in copious distinctly peduncled lax or dense racemes; bracts large, membraneous, ovate, caducous; pedicels short, densely pubescent. Corolla yellowish-red, 1/2 in. long calyx finally 1. 1 1/4 in., long, the scarious conspicuously veined lower lip 1 in. broad.

January to April, and other months.

Central Provinces, Western and Southern India and in Upper Burma. Madhya Pradesh, forests of North Oudh, Upper Gangetic Plains.

26.1 **Paracalyx sacriosa** (Roxb.) Ali. syn. *Cylista sacriosa* Roxb. Climbing tomentose undershrub. Leaf rachis up to 6 cm. long; leaflets rhomboid-ovate, acuminate, up to 5 X 4 cm., distinctly nerved beneath. Raceme 5-20 cm, long. Calyx up to 3 cm. long. Corolla yellow.

South India. Frequent in upper Ghats and plains, Karnataka, and other areas in southern region.

26.2 The type species of *Cylista* Aiton.is a member of the genus *Rhynchosia* Lour. suggesting necessity for a new generic name for the species of *Cylista* other than the type.

Rhynchosia tomentosa (Roxb.) *Cylista tomentosa* Roxb., *Rhynchosis cyanosperma* Benth.. It is woody climber, with white or red flowers; and native to Western Peninsular India, and is found under cultivation in some gardens (Siwalik or foot hills, Uttar Pradesh).

26.3 The plant *Cylista scariosa* Roxb. is medicinally useful

Roots are astringent and used in form of a decoction as a remedy for dysentery and leucorrhoea. Roots are also applied externally along with other drugs to reduce tumours.

Roots contain about 10% tannin.

The leaves of plant *Paracalyx scariosa* (Roxb.) All are considered an antidote in snake bite. Roots are useful in veneral diseases. Roots are useful as stomachic medicine. Leaves have vermicide properties and useful in worms affections.

27. ŚŪKAPARṆĀ-KṚṢYABHŪRUHĀ-PRASAVAPĪTĀ-STAMBHAMŪLADALĀ-NIRĀMAYĪ

S 27. Sonchus asper (Linn.) Hill.

Sonchus oleraceus (asper) Linn.

Asteraceae (Compositae)

Jalynniar, Akatsu

Erect, slender, simple or sparingly branched annual herbs, 15-100 cm. tall. Stems glabrous. Basal leaves in a rosette, petioled, spatulate-oblong, entire or pinnatifid to-partite, spinulosely dentate; cauline ones semi-amplexicaul, with rounded basal auricles, glabrous. Heads axillary, on 1-3 cm. long, gland-hairy peduncles, combined into a terminal sub-umbellate corymb, 1.1.3 cm. long. Involucral bracts 2 to 3-seriate, lanceolate, obtuse, glabrous except thinly gland-hairy; outer ones 0.5-1 cm. long. Corolla yellow, 1-1.3 cm. long. Achenes 3-ribbed on lateral faces, obovoid-oblong, with a thickened, serrate margin, 0.2-0.25 x 0.1 cm. Pappus-hairs, white, 1 cm. long.

Cold season; March to November

Widely distributed in India, and in the Himalayan regions up to 12,000 ft. elevation. China and many other temperate and tropical countries, but often introduced.

27.1 *Sonchus asper* Hill. syn. *S. oleraceous* Wall. An annual 2-3 ft. high, glabrous at sparsely glandular above, subumbellately branched. Leaves lanceolate cauline, 6-10 in. long, elliptic-oblong, entire, runciate or pinnatifid, 4-amplexicaul at the base, with round auricles entire or pinnatifidly toothed, auricles appressed, the margins undulate and dentate or spinous dentate. Heads crowded in umbel-like cymes, up to 1 in. diam. Involucral bracts glabrous. Achenes compressed, the faces 3-ribbed, nor or only faintly rugose between the ribs, or muricate between the ribs.

Upper Gangetic Plains and Siwalik range; Waste places, waysides, agricultural fields and other localities including cultivated place in various regions.

27.2 **Sonchus brachyotus** DC.

Sonchus arvensis auct. pl. (non Linn.)

Asteraceae

Erect, perennial herbs, with a thick, stout taproot, up to 5-80 cm. tall. Stems simple or sparingly branched in the upper part, glabrous, often pruinose. Basal leaves in a rosette; lower ones approximate; upper ones remote, oblong or spatulate-oblong, entire or lyrate-pinnatilobed, with a semi-amplexicaul base; basal auricles rounded, mucronate, shortly acutely dentate, pale beneath. Heads 1.5 cm. long on 1-5 cm. long, white-flocose, gland-bristly peduncles, combined, combined into branched corymbs. Involucral bracts 3 to 4-seriate, lanceolate, acute, 0.5-1 cm. long; outer ones white- flocose, densely clothed with gland-bristles. Corolla bright yellow, 1.5 cm. long; turning to brownish red on maturity. Achenes linear- oblong, curved, faintly transversely rugose, 5-ribbed on lateral faces, often alternating with intermediate ribs, 0.3 cm. long. Pappus-hairs white, 0.9-1 cm. long.

March to November, July to October.

Siwalik ranges, Dehadun, Uttar Pradesh.

27.3 **Sonchus arvensis** Linn.

Asteraceae

Perennial herb with a creeping and stoloniferous taptstock. Stems 2-4 ft. hollow, angular, umbellately branched and glanular-hairy above. Leaves mostly radical, runciate-pinnatifid, spinous-toothed; cauline amplexicaul with appressed rounded auricles; uppermost leaves linear. Heads few 1-2 in. diam., umbellately corymbose; peduncles and involucral bracts gland-hispid. Achenes narrow slightly compressed, prominently ribbed on each face and transeversely rugose. Pappus very white.

Cold season, July to October, October to February.

Sparingly throughout the plains of India, more abudant in the hills, ascending to 8,000 ft. elevation on the Himalayas. China and in most temperature in many tropical countries, either wild or introduced.

27.4 *Sonchus arvensis* Linn syh. *S. orixensis* Roxb. An annual milky herb with creeping rootstock, Leaves radical.

Sub-Himalayan tracts, Siwaliks, Dehradun, Uttar Pradesh *Sonchus arvensis* Linn. Herb glabrous towards the base, glandular hairy upwards; stems 2-4 ft. Leaves mostly radical, pinnatifid, 4-6 in.; lobes pointing downwards; teeth small; basis lobes rounded, appressed to the stem. Heads 1-2 in. diam.

Himachal Pradesh, Shimla, and other various areas; road-sides, common. Throughout India, (ascending to 8,000 ft.) All temperature and many tropical regions; Assam province, Khasi hills.

Sonchus arvensis Linn. syns. Sonchus wightianus DC; *S. orixensis* Roxb.; *S. wallichiana* DC.; *S. longifolia* Wall. Herb with creeping rootstock and glabrous tall stem, throughout India, wild in cutlivated places, scarce in the plains, common in the Khasia and Himalayas.

27.5 **Sonchus brachyotus** DC is hiterto referred *Sonchus arvensis* Linn.-An exclussively European species-but this is easily recognizable by shorter, narrower, fairly rugose achenes, shorter involucres, corolla, heads an pappus-hairs. *Sonchus arvensis* Linn. is characterized by transversely rugose, 0.4-0.45 cm., long achenes, 1.5 cm. long involucres, 2- 2.5 cm. long corollas and 2-2.5 cm. long heads and 1.5 cm. long, white pappus-hairs.

Sanchus brachyotes DC (*Sanchus arvensis* acuh. non Linn. sensu Hook, f.). An erect, succulent herb, glabrous towards the base, glandular hairy upwards. Leaves mostly radical pinnatifid, lobed pointing downwards, basal lobes rounded, appressed to the stem. Heads yellow; pappus white, ligules long. Achenes flattened and ovate.

Throughout India; Uttar Pradesh hills, Sub-Himalayan tracts, (ascending to 25.00 m.); wild and in cultivated place in different; regions; ravin slopes, water courses along lakes and ponds and field borders.

27.5 **Sonchus oleraceus** Linn.

Sonchus ciliatus Lamk.

S. royleanus Wall.

Asteraceae

Mahatama (Bombay), Titaliya (Bihar), Dodak (Punjabi), Ratrinta (Telague); chaker-patti.

Erect, simple or sparingly branches, annual herbs, 20-150 cm. tall. Stems fistular, glabrous in the lower part, gland-hairy upwards, often purple-tinged. Leaves oblong or obovate-oblong, with a sagitate base, acute, irregularly dentate, glaucous on the lower surface; lower ones narrowed into a petiole, painnatifid to-partite, with aciculate-dentate lobes. Heads 2 cm. across, on gland-hairy pedicels of 1-5 cm. long. Achenes transversely rugose, 3-ribbed on lateral faces, 0.3 X 0.1 cm. Pappus-hairs white, 0.5-0.6 cm. long.

July to October; February to May, post Cold season

Throughout India, ascending up to 8,000 ft. on the Himalayas. China and in many temperate and tropical countries; but often introduced.

27.7 **Sonchus oleraceus** Linn.

Erect, annual, 2-3 ft. high, glabrous or sparsely glandular-hispid. Stems subumbellately branched above, glaucous. Leaves thin, 6-10 in. long. lanceolate, entire or pinnatifid and with the terminal lobe large and the lateral lobes pointing downwards teeth small; the base sub-amplexicaul and with acute spreading auricles. Heads up to in in. in diam., arranged in umbellate cymes. Involucre bracts glabrous or nearly so. Achenes small, compressed, narrowly obvoid, the faces 3- ribbed and muriculate between the ribs.

Upper Gangetic Plains, abundant within the area especially on cultivated grounds.

27.8 **Sonchus oleraceus** Linn. A glabrous or slightly glandular herb on the upper parts. Stem branched. Leaves thin, lanceolate or pinnatifid; terminal leaves large, lateral lobes pointing downwards, sometimes only one pair; teeth small; basal lobes acute, entire or pinnatifid. Heads yellow. Achenes compressed, faces 3-ribbed and muricate between the ribs.

Siwalik range, foot hills, Dehradun, Uttar Pradesh; wild and in cultivated places, common in roadsides, waste places and agricultural fields and other localities.

27.9 **Sonchus wightianus** DC.

Sonchus arvensis auct. non L.

Dudoriban, Gyamatal-Ruzadara.

Herbs with creeping rootstock, up to 1.25 m.; terete, grooved, nearly glabrous. Leaves 10-30 X 2-5 m., oblong-lanceolate, acute-rounded at tip, cordate and amplexicaul at base, runcinate, galucous beneath. Heads in sparse panicles; bracts lanceolate, acute, outer bracts shorter, grandular hairy. Ligulate corollā up to 1.8 cm. long, bright yellow. Achenes minutely muricate.

August to May

Temperature to Tropics. Common but widely scattered in plains and upper Ghats. along readsides in moist, well-drained areas, Karnataka. Southern India.

27.10 *Sonchus maritimus* Linn. syn. *Sonchus arvonsis* Claarke. Punjab, Peswar, Westwards to the Atlantic.

Sonchus wightianus ash. *wallichianus* (DC.) Boulos.

Sonchus wallichianus DC.

S. arvensis var. *laevipes* auct. non Koch.

Sonchus wightianus DC. asp. *wightianus*

Sonchus arvensis such. non Linn.

Possibility is there about this species for not being distinct form *Sonchus arvensis* Linn.

27.11 Different species of *Sonchus* Linn. are distinguished on the basis of salient feature of plants. Outer involucral bracts desnely clothed with coarse gland-bristles, and achenes 0.3 cm. long perenniеal plants of *Sonchus brochotes* DC.; when involucral bracts without gland bristles, and achones 0.2-0.3 cm. in annual plants of other two species. They are distinguished by characters of achenes and basal auricles mainly. *Sonchus oleraceus* Linn. is with transversely rugose and thick achenes with a slightly thickened margins, acute leaves of basal auricles; whereas the achenes smooth, with a winged margin papery and basal auricles leaves rounded in *Sonchus asper* (Linn.) Hill.

Sanchus oleraceus Linn. and *Sonchus wightianus* DC. may also be broadly separated by deeply incised leaves in former, and leaves not incised in the latter species.

Moreover, the leaves are hard, teeth long, unequal and spinous in *Sonchus asper* Garasults; when the leaves thin, teeth small, prickly and not spinous in other two species which may be separated by basal lobes of stem leaves acute in *Sonchus oleraceus* Linn. whereas basal lobes of stem leaves rounded in *Sonchus brachyotes* DC.

Involucral bracts are gland-hair, achenes slightly compressed and transversely rugose in *Sonchus arvensis* Linn., which may be separated by *Sonchus asper* will having involucral bracts without gland-tipped hairs, and achenes much compressed, not transversely rugose.

27.12 Various species of *Sonchus* Linn. are medicinally useful, and utilised for other purposes. Plants of *Sonchus cleracous* Linn are useful as fodder for cattles. Similarly the cattels are very fond of eating the plants of *Sonchus arvensis* Linn.

The roots of *Sonchus arvensis* Linn. are given in jaundice. Seeds are considered demulcent. Medicinal properties are almost similar to *Lactuca serriola* Linn. Plant is cooling, sedative, diuretic, diaphoretic, antispasmodic and expectorant.

Plant contains bitter principles.

Medicinal properties and uses of *Sonchus maritimus* Linn. are considered similar to *S. arvensts* and *Lactuca* species.

Plant of *Sonchus asper* Hill. is pounded and applied to wounds and boils as external application.

Plant contains bitter substance.

The gum formed by evaporation of the juice of the plant of *Sonchus oleraceus* Linn. is considered a powerful hydragogue cathartic. Infusion of roots and leaves is used as tonic and febrifuge, and used in fevers.

Leaves are galactogogue, febrifuge and cholagogue. They are used in juindice, fever, and other ailments. Latex is used in liver complaints. Leaves are useful as tonic and used in general debility.

Whole plant of *Sonchus wightianus* DC syn. *S.arvensis* Hk. is useful in cholera. Herb and leaves are applied in cuts and wounds. Whole plant is in useful dysentery. Plant is edible as vegetable.

Stem of *S. asper* Linn. is also edible as vegetable.

28. MAHĀLATĀ-CATUṢVARTIKĀGRĪ-AṄG-ULIPATRAKA-CATUṢṬAYĪPUṢPA-AVRAṆĀ

P 28. **Tetrastigma campylocarpum** (Kurz.) Planch.

Tetrastigma campylocarpa Kurz.

Vitis campylocarpa Kurz.

V. parkeri Gangepain.

Vitaceae

Tasram-doukha (Kachar), Bepui-rhui (Lushai).

Large evergreen climber with stems up to 22 cm. in diam. and 27 meters high. Stems terete. Bark reddish-brown. Very rough and rather corky, furrowed and often deeply se. Blaze very fibrous, pink or white streaked with pink turning orange on exposure, very shiny and turning purplish black on the blade of a knife. Tendrils simple, often short and long. Twigs small, green, glabrous, without prominent lenticels. Leaves digitately 3-6-0.5 cm., swollen, Terminal leaflets 4-7 by 2.5-4 cm. elliptic, abruptly acuminate, often caudate, glabrous, rather thick, dark somewhat shining green above, paler and shining beneath, lateral nerves 3-4 paris, arcuate; lateral pair of leaflets smaller. petiolule of terminal leaflets, 0.5-1.75 cm. long, of the lateral shorter. Flowers polygamodioeceous, 4-merous, in lax, rather slender, puberulous, subcorymbose, axiliary cymes. Fruit 0.4-0.8 cm. long, oblong or ovoids first reddish and finally black. seeds 1-3, usually 1, ellipsoid. 0.3-0.5 cm. long with 6-10 shallow transverse furrows.

November to December, March to May.

Assam province; fairly common in the evergreen forests in Upper Assam and Surman valley in hilly vicinities. Uttar Pradesh, Siwaliks and Terai region.

28.1 **Tetrastigma serrulatum** (Roxb.) Planch

Cissus serrulata Roxb.

Vitis capreolata D. Den.

V. affine Gangep. ex Osmasten.

Tetrastigma affine (Osmasten) Raizada & Saxena

T. indicum Maulik.

Vitaceae

Slender, glabrous climbers, with simple or forked tendrils. Leaves digitately 5-foliolate; leaflets subsessile, obovate-lanceolate, cuneate at hase, acute-subacuminate at apex, serrate-denticulata. Petiole. 2-8 (.10) cm. long. Flowers in umbellate clusters. Berry 0.5-0.8 cm. across.

August to September, October to November.

Uttar Pradesh, Siwaliks and also terai region; plant in ravines and rocky of river banks, scattered or varrying fequency.

28.2 **Tetrastigma thomsonianum** Planch.

Tetrastigma augustifolia (Roxb.) Deb.

Vitis angustifolia (Roxb.) W.

non **T. angustifolia** Planch

Vitaceae

Netung-riubi (Miri-Assam).

Herbaceous climber with dark-coloured usually flattened stems. Leaves 3-foliolate, common petiole 2-3 in. long, glabrous; stipules ovate-oblong, about 15-20 in. long, coriaceous. Leaflets 3-6 by 1-1.5 in., lanceolate or elliptic-lanceolate, distantly serrate, acuminate, glabrous or puberulous on the midrib; main lateral nerves 5-7 on either half, slender. Tendrils simple, leaf-opposed, very slender. Cymes axillary, short or-shorter than the common petiole, dense usually very shortly peduncled, subescent. Flowers 4-merous, dioeceous, green; Petals free. Sytle 0.; stigma large, flat, scarcely lobed. Berry globose about .2 in. across, not juicy, 2-4 seeded. Seeds furrowed on each face and transeversely rugose on the sides.

September to October; December to January.

Plant not uncommon in the islands, and along the banks of the Brahmaputra; also in Sylhet and Khasi hills.

28.3 **Tetrastigma obtectum** (Wall ex Lawson) Planch.

Vitis obtecta Wall ex Lawson.

Vitasceae

Evergreen climber creeping over the surface of the ground of climbing up the stems of trees to which it closely adheres by means of tendrils and numerous adventitious roots, the stem attaining 40 ft. height and 1 in. diam., but usually half this height. Tendrils consisting of a stout stalk .1-.25 in. long terminating in 5-9 palmately rediating simple spirally coiled branches. 5-1.5 in. long which develop adhesive disks on contract. Leaves digitately 5-foliolate. Petiole 1.5-5 in. long, torete, pinkish, clothed with spreading pale hairs. Terminal leaflets pinkish, clothed with spreading pale hairs. Terminal leaflets ellipitc, 2-4 by 1.25 in. with about 5-8; pairs of lateral neves; Petiolutes of terminal leaflets 0-.25 in. long. Flowers small, green, 4-merous, in few branched pubescent cymes. the branches terminating in umbels. Fruits .3-.5 in. diam. elliptic or globose, shining black. Seeds. 1-2.

May to June; October to November.

Plant occurring throughout the Kumash hilly region, Uttar-Pradesh hills between 4,500 to 7,000 fit.; common in shady forests and moist ravines especially in banj forests.

Some other species of Tetrastigma may be referred relevanily.

28.4 **Tetrastigma bracteolatum** (Wall.) Planch

Vitis bracteolata Wall.

- **T. canarense** (Dalz.) Gamble.

V. canarensis Dalz.

T. dubium (Lawson) Planch.

- **V. dubia** Lawson.

T. hookeri (Lewson) Planch

- **V. hookeri** Lawson.

T. obovatum (Lawson) Gengip.

- **V. obovata** Lawson.

T. obtectum (Wall. ex Lawson) Planch.

- **V. obtecta** Wall. ex Lawson.

T. thomsonianum Planch.

- **T. angustifolia** (Roxb.) Deb.
- **V. angustifolia** (Hoxb.) Wall.

28.5 *Vitis parkeri Gagnepain.* A large evergreen climber with stems up to 9 in. diam. and 80 ft. high. stems terete. Bark reddish-brown, very rough and rather corky, furrowed and often deeply sp. Blaze very fibrous, pink or white streaked with pink turning purplish black on the blade of a knife. Tendrils simple, often about and long. Twigs smooth, green, glabrous, without the prominent-lenticels. Leaves digitately 3-6-foliolate, not pedate (never), on 4-8 in. petiole, with, 5 in. swollen basal. Terminal leaflets elliptic, abruptly acuminate often caudate, rather thick, dark somewhat shining green above, paler and shining beneath. Petiolules of terminal leaflets. 5-1.75 in. long of the lateral shorter. Flowers small, 4-merous, in lax, rather slender, puberulous, subcorymbose, axillary cymes. Fruits oblong or ovoid, initially reddish turning black, with 1-3 seeds (usually 1), ellipsoid, shallow transversely furrowed.

Plant fairly common in sal forests between 1,500 and 3,000 ft. especially in moist ravines and on the banks of shady streams, in Kumaon region, Uttar Pradesh Hills; throughout the Sub-Himalayan tract and outer hill rages. It comes in flowering stage during November to December, and bears fruits in April to May months.

28.6 Presently *Tetrastigma campylocarpun* (Kurz.) Planch, *Vitis campylocarpa* Kurz., *T. parkeri* Gagnepain are treated synonymous, carrying previous similarity and distinctions based on observations by some authorities on different plants representing various areas of occurrence of *Tetrabtigma* species in particular and allied plants.

28.7 Tetrastigma leucostaphylum (Dennst.) Alston.

Tetrastigma muricatum (Wight. & Arn.) Gamble

Vitis muricata Wall ex. Wight & Arn.

V. leucostaphyla (D.) Jacksno.

V. lanceolaria sensu Lausa Cissus leucostaphyla Dennst.

Vitaceae

Climbers. Brranchs terete, muricate. Leaves usually 3-foliolate; leaflets 10-15 X 5-8 cm., broadly elliptic, rounded at base, distantly serrate. Inflorescence branches ferruginous, rarely glabrate. flowers greenish-white. Calyx and petals hairy. Berry up to 1 cm. acress.

December to February.

South-Western India. Plant common in semi-evergreen forests in lower Ghats, Karnataka.

28.8 **Tetrastima sulcatum** (Lawson) Gamble.

Vitis sulcata Bawson.

Vitaceae

Climbers. Branches angled, sulcate. Leaves 3-4-foliolate; leaflets 6-9 X 2-4 cm., elliptic; lateral leaflets asymmetric Inflorescence bunches hairy. Fruit 2.2.5 cm. across.

February to March, or spring season.

South-Western India. Plant eccasional in wet deciduous to semi-evergreen forests in Ghats, Karnataka. Madras state (Tamilnadu) and other regions in southern region.

28.9 Tetrastigma Planchon, formerly included under *Vitis* Linnaeus, is resultant of division later and with petals 4, stigmas nearly sessile, 4-lobed and inflorescence axillary as the salient characters in member species.

28.10 Tetrastigma lanceolarium Planchen.

Vitis lanceolaria Wall ex Wight.

Cissus lancelaria Roxb.

Tetrastigma lanceoarium (Roxb.) Planch.

Vitaceae

Tadi-ripun-riubi (Miri).

Large woody evergreen, glabrous, climbers; stems, branchlets and petioles often corky-tubercled, tendrils simple, glabrous. Leaves pedately, 5-foliolate, those of coppice shoots often 3-foliolate; leaflets lanceolate or ovate/lanceolate, distantly serrate, 3-5 in. long. Flowers unisexual, pale yellow, tetramerous, stigma 4-lobed. Cymes axillary, dichotomously compound, peduncles short, the female cymes smaller, petals distinct. Fruits 1/2 in. diam.

February to April.

Nepal, Oudh Forests. Uttar Pradesh hilly region (Kumaon), Sikkim (ascending to 4,000 ft.), Sylhet, Manipur. Western Ghats from North Canara southwards; Andamans Islands. Lower Burma.

28.11 **Tetrastigma rumicispermum** Lawson) Planchon.

Vitis rumicispermum Lawson.

V. rumicisperma Law.

Vitaceae

Large glabrous climber. Branches covered with corky tubercles, Cymes compound, dichotomous, simple, langer than common petiole. Fruits edible; seeds broadly triangular keeled.

Eastern Himalayan region; Sikkim (5-7, 000 ft. elevations), Khasi hills. Manipur.

28.12 Various species of *Tetrastigma* Planchon are medicinally useful and also a few used in allied purposes including edible and vegetable items from herbal sources.

The poultice of leaves of the plant *Tetrastigma lanceolarium* Planch. is made and applied to boils, and also to the body for ague.

The leaves of *Tetrastigma lanceolarium* (Roxb.) Planch. are useful in fever.

The fruits of the plant are edible.

The leaves and twigs of the plant *Tetrastigma leucophyllum* (Dennst) Alston. syn. *T. muricatum* Planch. are edible and employed for cooking vegetable and eaten. This plant is known as Moja-hei and other names in different regions. The leaves of the plant *Tetrastigma serrulata* (Roxb.) Planch. syn. *Vitis capreolata* Don. are ground and made a paste which applied to boils, wounds and ulcers.

The fruits of the plant *Tetrastigma rumicispermum* (Laws.) plant are edible.

Tetrastigma lanceolarium (Roxb.) Planch. Syn. *Vitis lanceolariam* Wall ex Wight & Arn, known as Bherseri (Nepal) and fundoror-rik (Lepcha) is medicinally useful. The fruits are eaten raw or cooked with fish. The leaves are much esteemed as sorrel. The poultice of the leaves are considered useful for applying to boils. The juice of the plant is used in cough.

Intergeneric grafting between grape and this species is reported to be possible. It is large climber evergreen, ascending to 18 meters, found in Kumaon to Sikkim and North Bengal, and in eastern and the peninsular India up to an alt. of 3,000 meters.

T. sarrulatum Planch. syn. *V. capreolata* D. Don, known as Charchari (Napal) is a beautiful climber with selender stems, often developing adventitious roots, found from Garhwal to Bhutan and in most parts of eastern India up to an alt. of 2,600 meters. The fruits are edible. The alcoholic extract of the aerial parts of the plant, when given intramuscularly, showed anticancer activity against Walker carcinosarcoma, 256 in rats. The plant is toxic to adult albino mica.

I. bracteolatum (Wall. ex ex M. Lawa) pianch syn. *V. bracteolata* Wall., known as soh-mei-boit (Khasi), Durujedoukhu (Cachar) and pundor-rik (Lspcha) is a handsome vine, found from Bihar end East Nepal to Bhutan and in eastern India up to an alt. of 600 meters, also occurring in Orissa and Andhra Presesh. *I. rumicispermum* (M. Laws) Planch syn. *V. rumicisperma* M. Laws is a very large climber, found from East Nepal to Sikkim-North Bengal, Arunachal Pradesh, Assam and Meghalaya, at alts. of 900-2, 400 meters. The fruits of both these species are eaten.

T. thomsonianum Planch syn. *V. angustifolia* Wail ex Wight. is a herbaceous climber with dark-coloured and ususally flattened stems and bright-red berries, found in Bihar, North Bengal, Assam, Meghalaya and Manipur. The tender stems and leaves are acidic, and are eaten cooked with fish.

T. canarensa (Dalz) gamble syn. *V. canarensis* Doiz. is an elegant climber with red or cadmium-yellow fruits, found in western Ghats up to 909 meters. The barries are eaten by the monkeys.

Selected Bibliography

Anonymous : Medicinal plants of India, Vol. I, ICMR, New Delhi 1976.

Anonymous : The Wealth of India (Raw Materials), Vols. 1-8, CSIR, New Delhi, 1948-69.

Babu, C.R. : Herbaceous Flora of Dehradun, CSIR, New Delhi, 1977.

Bennet, S.S.R, Name Changes in Flowering Plants of India and Adjacent Regions, Dehradun, 1987.

Brandis, D. : Indian Trees, London, 1931

Brandis, D. : The forest Flora of North-West and Central India, Landon, 1874.

Chopra, R.N. et al : Glossary of Indian Medicinal Plants, CSIR, New Delhi, 1956.

Chopra, R.N. Supplement to G.I.M.P., CSIR, New Delhi, 1969

Chopra, R.N. Indigenous Drugs of India, 2nd. ed., Calcutta, 1958

Chopra, R.N. Poisonous Plants of India, 2 vols., New Delhi 1965

Collett, N. : Flora Simlensis, Calcutta, 1921.

Cooke, T. : Flora of Bombay, Vols, 1-3, BSI, Calcutta, Rept. 1960

Duke, J.A. : Isthmian Ethnobotanical Dictionary, Jodhpur, 1981.

Duthie, J. F. : Flora of Upper Gangetic Plains, Vols. 1-2, BSI, Calcutta, Rept. 1960.

Gamble, J. S. : Flora of Madras, London, Vols. 1-3, 1915-36.

Haines, H.H. : Botany of Bihar and Orissa, Vols. 1-3, BSI Calcutta, Rept. 1861.

Hooker, J. D. : Flora of British India, Vols. 1-7, London, 1872-97.

Jain, S.K. : Dictionary of Indian Folk Medicine and Ethonobotany, New Delhi, 1991.

Kanjilal, U. N. et al : Flora of Assam, Vols. 1-5, Shillong, 1935.

Kirtikar, K. R. et al : Indian Medicinal Plants, Vols. 1-4, Allahabad, 1933.

Maheshwari, J.K. : The Flora of Delhi, CSIR, New Delhi, 1963.

Osmasten, A. F. : Forest Flora of Kumaon, Allahabad, 1927.

Pandey, Gyanendra : Puspayurveda-Medicinal Flowers of India and adjacent regions, Delhi. 1992.

Pandey, Gyanendra : Gyanendra Enumeratio Plantamedica (Editor Sumitra Pandey), Delhi, 1993.

Pandey, Gyanendra Vanoushadhi Manjusha-Maidani Ksetron Ki Upayogi Vanaspatiyan, (by Prof. Ram Nath Vaidya), Hardwar, 1990.

Pandey, Gyanendra : Uncommon plant Drugs of Ayurveda, Delhi, 1993.

Pandey, Gyanendra : Medicinal Plants of Himalaya, Vol. I, Delhi, 1995.

Parkinson, C.E.A. : Forest Flora of the Andamans Islands, Simla, 1923.

Prain, D. : Bengal plants, Calcutta, Vols. 1-2, 1903.

Raizada, M.R. : Supplement to Duthie's Flora of Upper Gangetic Plains, Dehradun, 1978.

Saldanha C. J. et al : Flora or Hassan District, Karnataka, India New Delhi, 1976.

Santapau, H. et al : A Dictionary of the Flowering plants of India, CSIR, New Delhi 1973.

Watt, G. : A Dictionary of Economic Products of India, 1908.

General Index

BOTANICAL NAMES